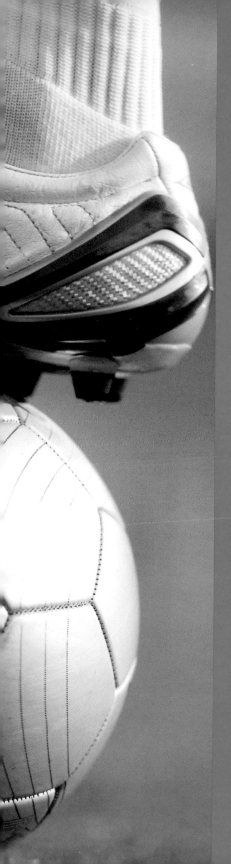

contents

foreword

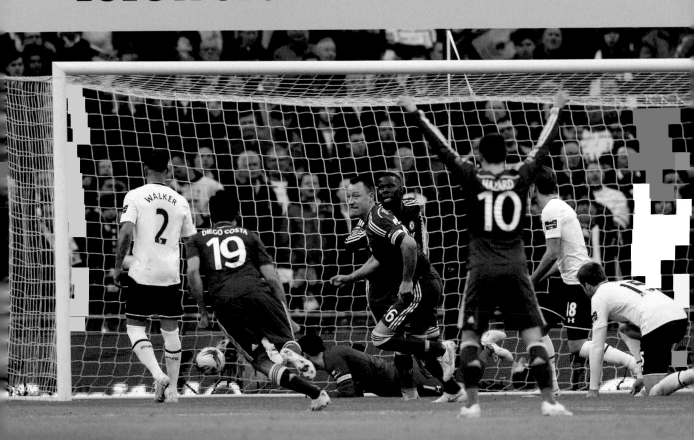

The modern game of football has never been faster, more dynamic or more entertaining to watch. This can be attributed to the influx of funding from television revenue in the last 20-25 years. Increased cash has increased research into the sport and the amount of expertise clubs can afford to employ in the search for an edge in winning matches. These range from specialist coaches, psychologists, nutritionists, and varied medical expertise to video and data analysts.

One of the areas to have enjoyed the biggest rise in influence in this time is strength and conditioning. As our understanding about football performance has grown we have come to understand the nuanced and widely diverse physical skill set the modern player must possess to perform optimally as well as the variation that is presented throughout the different positions in a team.

This has led to a virtuous cycle whereby players get fitter and the demands of the game increase, asking yet more of the players and support staff. Although not always considered so, the modern elite player is also an elite athlete. They must be able to run and sprint repeatedly with unknown rest periods, jump high, be strong in the air and hold opposition players off the ball as well as pass and shoot the ball regularly with power. All of these attributes test the capacity of the player's strength, endurance, flexibility and mobility. Weaknesses in any one of these areas can affect team performance, directly and indirectly. Performance can be directly affected when a central defender is pushed off the ball by a striker in the box who goes on to score. Team performance can be affected indirectly when a player tears a hamstring and misses the next 4-6 weeks of games.

However the base physical skills and movements of the game do not change from a Sunday morning league game to the World Cup final, only the intensity with which they are performed. It is not sufficient therefore for any player, serious about their performance (and avoiding injury) to not consider specific work in these areas. Strangely though it is one area that is often forgotten or missed out away from the professional level where players have coaches to plan their work for them. Fortunately now this book (amazingly one of the first published in this sector) presents the techniques and plans for success from one of the leaders in the field, and is bang up to date with some of the latest thinking and expertise. It should be considered essential reading for players of any age who aspire to greatness, whether that be on the world stage or in the local park.

Jack Nayler, First Team Sports Scientist/Conditioning Coach at Real Madrid C.F.

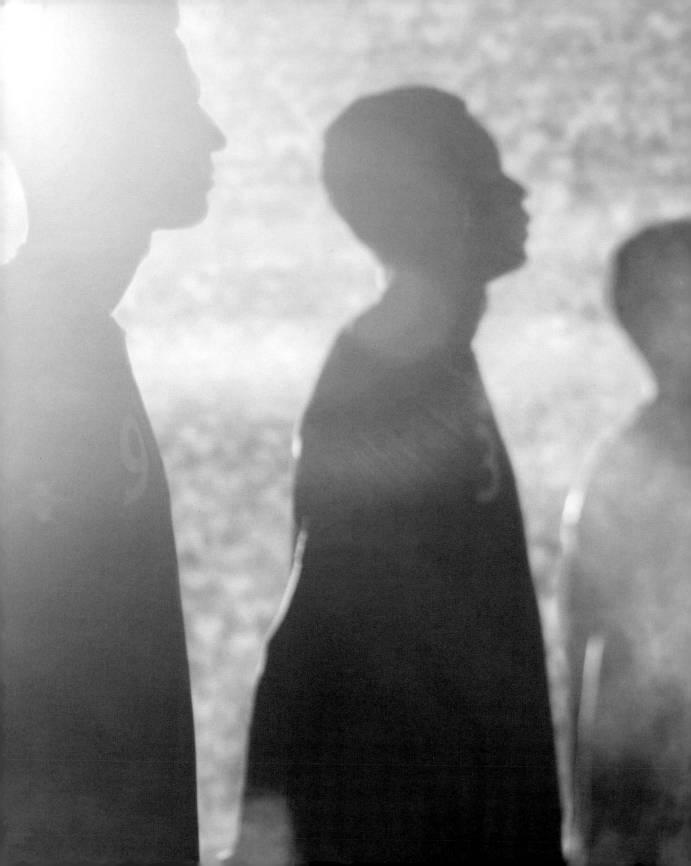

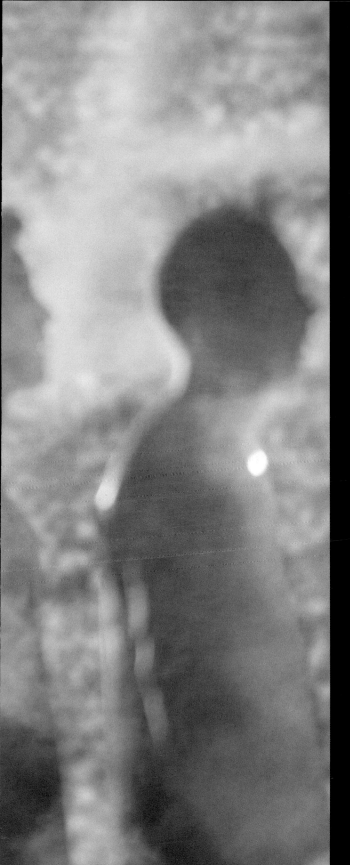

part 1

philosophy and effective practice

001
introduction

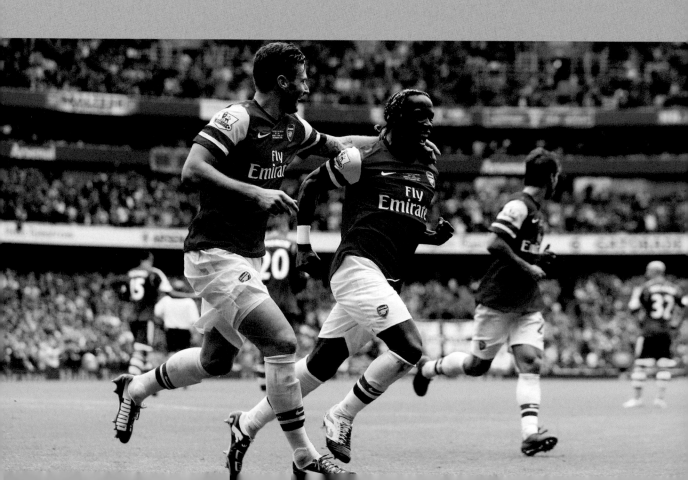

1.1 A History of Strength and Conditioning in Football – A Rocky Relationship

The concept of a specialist strength and conditioning (S&C) coach is still a relatively new one. The first cohort of coaches with an S&C job title didn't emerge in the UK until the early 2000s. Of course, professional football has utilised S&C for decades – it just wasn't called that. This came in many forms and was delivered from all kinds of sources. Most commonly it would have come from the fitness coach, who has become known as the sports scientist in recent years. However, physios, coaches and even players with some degree of gym experience have all been known to deliver.

The genesis of the fitness coach into a sports scientist is key to the emergence of the S&C specialist. Many years ago the fitness coach, typically an ex-player, would be responsible for the warm-up and 'running the lads'. As a Jack-of-all-trades he would also dispense casual dietary advice and maybe even spot the odd set of bench press. As sports science has grown, the range of responsibilities simply makes genuine expertise in each of these areas impossible. The processing and interpretation of the mass of data generated by heart-rate and GPS data, both now standard practice in the professional game, is practically a full-time job alone. The basics of nutrition can be covered but again, a specialist is required to solve individual support at the highest level. And finally S&C. Providing bespoke, precise and expert programming and coaching to achieve targeted goals in an elite player requires a specialist. It is for this reason that I despair when I see jobs advertised as Sports Scientist/S&C Coach – using the term simply due to its fashionable status.

In many ways, the job title of the person delivering S&C is irrelevant. After all, job titles and qualifications are neither proof of quality, nor are their absence proof of inadequacy. What is more of a problem is the lack of consensus as to exactly what S&C can offer or what it is there to achieve. I have never been a big fan of the term 'strength and conditioning', and have personally found that it is frequently a barrier to understanding with coaches from a variety of sports. Specifically, the word 'strength' tends to subconsciously induce a fear that the aim is to produce muscle-bound powerhouses. This is compounded by decades of misconceptions as to the purpose of weights as a training tool. The association with body-building is still an issue today.

What's more, there are many routes to success on the football pitch. While some players rely on strength and speed to dominate the opponent, others rely on technique and ability to read the game. Sceptics of gym training are all too quick to point out examples of excellent players who rely on the latter (e.g. Iniesta and Xavi), or even those who are blessed with a physique that allows them to be physically dominant without additional work (e.g. Lukaku and Drogba). Of course, common sense tells us that this simply means that we can only state that S&C *may* help your game, rather than insisting that it *will*. Sadly, the subtleties of such arguments are rarely given much airtime when discussing with a coach or player who has decided they don't want to walk through the door.

In fairness it should be acknowledged that S&C coaches in almost every sport have had to overcome these issues. We have all had to prove our worth as the profession becomes more established and the understanding of the full breadth of what good S&C can offer emerges.

One of my key aims in this book is to lay down a philosophy as to how I believe S&C can add genuine value to professional football. However, I must also stress that this is very much a philosophy rather than an unquestionable set of rules. There will be coaches who I'm sure disagree with some of my assertions and pursue an alternative philosophy. That is fine, and is part of the joy of our profession. There are many routes to success, and the fact that we all solve the puzzle in a slightly different way makes it all the more interesting. If by committing my philosophy to text and sharing with colleagues I can help to cement our understanding and move the debate forward, then it will have been entirely worthwhile.

1.2 Defining Our Terms

I've already spoken of the confusion that can be caused by the term S&C, and so before we go any further it's important that we are clear exactly what we are talking about.

In general I think the best and most concise definition of S&C is: 'the physical preparation of athletes'. There are a few points to note here. There is no mention of the level of athlete – it still counts as S&C in non-elite athletes. In my view though, it is directed towards athletic *performance*. Personal trainers may use S&C tools, and may be very effective and knowledgeable, but training for general health or aesthetics is not S&C in my view. The other point to note is that the definition is intentionally broad in that no limits are placed on what the training process may involve. In general this is key, as the S&C coach should be holistic in his thought process and use whichever tools and methods will prove most effective. We are defined by our goals, not our methods.

So, with such a broad definition available to us, surely all elements of a player's training fall under the remit of S&C? Maybe, but that is not how we will treat the role in this book. If for no other reason, the time required to give due attention to a squad of players makes it unfeasible for one person to deliver high quality in both on-field conditioning and gym work. Not only is the task too large, but also logistically it is almost impossible. If some players require or request additional conditioning after the main session, how can the coach also be available for post-training gym work? Similarly, if the outside warm-up is being prepared, how can that person be indoors coaching individualised preparatory work?

At this point I should acknowledge that there are high-profile practitioners who have attempted this challenge, albeit with significant support from assistant S&C coaches. Credit goes to them for exceptional organisational skills but I believe they are the exception, and would possibly venture that they could have been more effective by not spreading themselves so thin.

My next point may upset a few readers, but if that is the collateral damage to moving our profession forward then it is an acceptable attrition. I believe that to be truly expert, not just very good but expert, we must dedicate ourselves to mastery of either the on-field conditioning or the supplementary work performed in the gym and rehab environment. Many will be reluctant to accept this. This is understandable, as we all generally have good knowledge of both and enjoy the variety. Consider what we know of expertise though. It is widely accepted that there is a strong relationship between expertise and the duration of study or exposure. If we invest in the concept of the S&C expert, this person has twice the time available to develop their craft and understanding as the coach who is splitting their role. It is hard to argue that this will not result in a higher level of coaching and insight.

It is for these reasons, and the fact that a wealth of literature describing methods of developing on-field training regimes is available, that within this text the term S&C refers to the supplementary training methods used to increase robustness and enhance performance.

1.3 My Journey

As I've already stated, much of this book is about a philosophy of S&C in football rather than a categorical definitive text. Consequently it is important to describe the journey that I took to form this philosophy.

Prior to my work in Premier League and Champions League football, I'd been fortunate enough to have been exposed to a huge variety of athletes in my work with Olympic and Paralympic sport at the English Institute of Sport. This has given me the opportunity to experiment with all types of training on athletes with different lifestyles, mentalities, and physical attributes. It was also a relatively safe environment to experiment in as, while results were always important, the major judgement comes every four years at the Olympics and Paralympics. This is in stark contrast to the week-to-week judgements under the harshest magnifying glass that is found in football.

It is this high-pressure, constantly changing environment which can make football so exciting to work in. Sadly though, it is not always the best place to develop your practice. When results aren't going well it often doesn't serve the S&C coach to start doing anything experimental. It is often he who puts his head above the parapet who will be first in the firing line if heads need to roll. My view has always been that the team winning games does not necessarily mean you've done a good job, but it may mean that you now have the chance to start doing one.

As a result of this need to watch your back, it is often the case that coaches seek to assimilate rather than innovate. Players reinforce this culture as they have an expectation of how their training will look. Anything outside the norm is often regarded as either a reflection of not knowing how to do things 'properly', or even worse, being 'busy'. (NB: 'busy' is a term commonly used in British football which refers to anyone being over the top and too keen – it's a very destructive concept as it discourages innovation and experimentation.) Often the only way around this is to come in with some level of guru status, and then the freedom may be granted to do things differently. For those working their way up from the bottom though, this can be a real barrier to technical progression.

This may seem to paint a very negative view of the football environment. I must stress that this is a general portrait of some of the common issues in the sport. These issues are neither ubiquitous nor non-negotiable. There are undoubtedly some pioneering thinkers, world-class practitioners, and open minded and insightful players and coaches. However, these issues still remain very real for a large proportion of those in the game.

In my experience, an expert tends to use his tools more sparingly than the keen novice who wishes to deploy them at every opportunity. It is easy to convince yourself that everything is a nail when you have just had a hammer lesson. My work in track and field in particular has afforded me a great opportunity to learn about the development of speed, strength and power. Critically, this has taught me not only how to use these tools but also to understand their limitations. Consequently I am comfortable using them sparingly. This will be discussed in much greater detail later, but I have found that even with Olympic level power athletes the greatest gains still come from helping them to move more effectively, rather than simply increasing their capacity to produce force. The powerful draw of football is such that many working in the game have not had this type of broad apprenticeship. Generally, their training will have included elements of strength and power such as Olympic lifts (e.g. power cleans, jerks, etc.) and plyometrics. It is only natural that there is a strong desire to put this learning into practice when working with players … regardless of whether this really is the best route to affecting performance. When discussing performance enhancement I will aim to expand upon general understanding of the use of these tools in football. I would encourage a more sparing, but ultimately more effective, integration of them into football S&C practice.

1.4 How to Use this Book

It is important to be aware that this is a text that aims to deal specifically with the questions, concerns and solutions involved in being effective in football. We will not cover the basics of anatomy and physiology and go over the fundamentals of S&C. These have been done elsewhere very well,

and so a shallow repetition would add nothing and only detract from being able to focus on the nuances of football. Therefore this is best combined with a good broad reading base. Personally I would recommend a number of texts and, of course, books should only form a portion of your education. If you are looking for somewhere to start I would recommend those in Table 1.1.

I should also be clear about the type of player this philosophy is aimed at. This is primarily coaches and players involved in the upper echelons of the game who have time to engage in specialist S&C. Part-time coaches are more likely to utilise their time on the training pitch, as are non-full-time players. However, many of the principles discussed here apply to novice just as well as elite. Indeed, they often apply to junior players too. The reason for this is that S&C training, age and technical ability do not relate to football ability. It is entirely possible for a part-time player to out-perform a Premier League player in the gym. Football is not a sport where we are required to fulfil our genetic potential in any one quality (in contrast to physiology dominant sports such as cycling or

Table 1.1	Recommended Supplementary Reading
Starting Strength, Mark Rippetoe, Aasgaard Company, 2007	
Becoming a Supple Leopard, Kelly Starrett, Victory Belt Publishing, 2013	
Anatomy Trains, Thomas Myers, Churchill Livingston, 2013	
Diagnosis & Treatment of Movement Impairment Syndromes, Shirley Sahrmann, Mosby, 2010	
Strength and Conditioning – Biological Principles and Practical Applications, Marco Cardinale, Human Kinetics, 2010	
Running: Biomechanics and Exercise Physiology in Practice, Frans Bosch, Churchill Livingston, 2004	
Ultimate Back Fitness & Performance, Stuart McGill, McGill, 2004	

sprinting). Equally, it is far from unknown for a high-level player to have learnt to cope with significant movement dysfunction and imbalance.

Anyone who has worked with any more than a handful of players will know that not all of them make an immediate connection between the gym and the pitch. Consequently, engagement in sessions is often less than 100%. A key feature of this book is that we will give significant airtime to the challenge of being an effective coach and how to 'bring players with you'. This is rarely given much consideration in S&C textbooks, where the focus tends to be solely on the technical content. However, in reality it is rarely the exercises on the programme that are the limiting factor in progress, but instead, the coach's ability to sell their message.

Just as the effective coach needs to think about more than 'just the programme', they also need an understanding of how their practice integrates with the 'big picture'. A classic mistake in junior S&C coaches is a failure to understand that their job is to SUPPORT the programme, not BE the programme. The mature coach must recognise that their goals overlap with others', and they must interact effectively if they are to be successful.

We've already established that this book doesn't aim to be the definitive text – it can't be, as football S&C is still on a journey. Rather it is a philosophy which is evidence-based, some from the literature, some from experience and years of practical application. A combination of these is crucial. Practical experimentation is vital if we are to push the boundaries of performance but equally we must be robust in our science and principles. This is summed up nicely by the popular schematic illustrated above. With that in mind I sometimes make suggestions for things that may work but we don't as yet know for sure (but I will always be clear

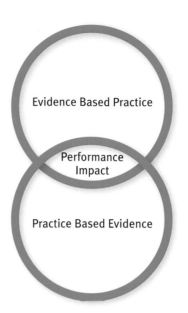

Figure 1.1 Achieving Performance Impact

to state this). Although some specifics in terms of training protocols and methodologies are given, these are often just to provide an example; this certainly isn't an S&C recipe book. I would much rather try to teach how to think and approach problems rather than just giving answers.

Not all of the questions around performance and training will be answered in these pages, but that is precisely the point. It is as important to pose new questions as it is to provide answers to the existing ones. In football we are often constrained by political balancing and practical limitations. The discussions in this book will hopefully give the S&C coach the opportunity to think in a space beyond their operational constraints.

In summary, I hope to move things forward and lay down a landmark in clearly defining exactly how S&C coaches can impact on the success of a top-level team. I hope you enjoy.

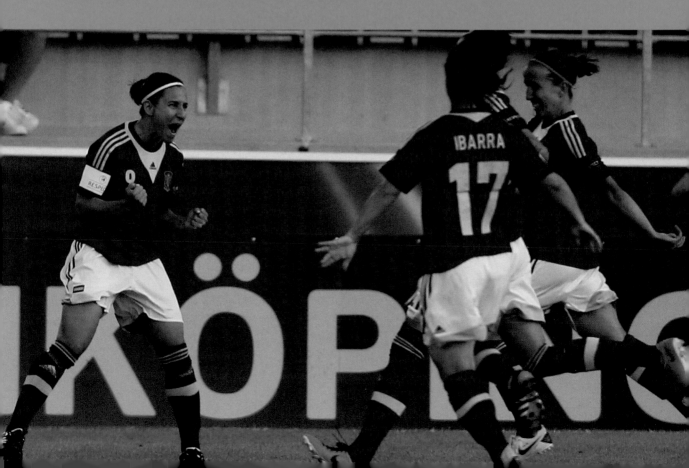

002
team sport
performance model

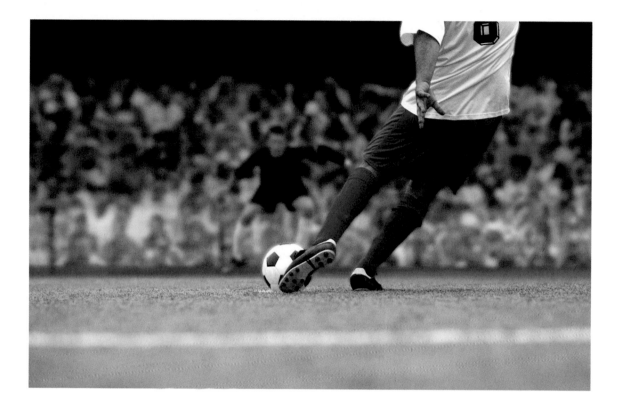

The 3rd, 4th and 6th categories in the performance model (**team balance**, **tactics** and **character**) clearly represent areas which S&C has no influence over. This alone is worth taking note of, as it should act as a stark reminder that we have no opportunity to affect at least 50% of the critical determinants of winning. What is more, the opposition must account for 50% of the result and so even on our best day we can only influence 25% of the result! A good cause for humility.

To my mind one of the biggest barriers sports scientists in football are yet to overcome is nailing down exactly what their key performance indicators (KPIs) are. Some sports lend themselves to this type of analysis much more naturally. For example, when working with a 100m sprinter it is too simplistic to merely focus on the finish time.

Coaches will break the race down and consider components such as reaction time, drive phase, stride length, peak velocity, etc. These can each be targeted with specific training strategies and, importantly, clearly have a direct effect on the overall performance. This means there is a clear link between the training, the KPI, and the result. The clear linking of these elements is illustrated in Figure 2.2 below.

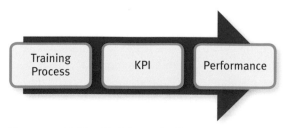

Figure 2.2 Linking Training to Performance

So what would be our KPIs for football? First of all let's please be clear that the result of the game should not be considered a KPI. I shouldn't need to say that, but I still find it amazing how many people are happy to assume that the team's success means that they are doing a good job. Of course you will hopefully have made a contribution, but there are countless factors which will have influenced the result to the point where this cannot be considered accountability. One thing top-level football is not lacking is things which can be measured. An ocean of data on physical statistics (distance covered, number of sprints, etc.), as well as technical metrics (possession, shots, etc.), are produced for every match. Frustratingly though, none of these provide us with the clear link from training to KPI to result which other sports enjoy. We know that if we are fitter we have the capacity to cover more distance. But as any intelligent player will tell you, the art of football is to run around the least, not the most! It certainly doesn't guarantee wins. While the significance of possession varies according to the style of the team, shots on target are perhaps the most telling technical metric. The only problem with this is that we can't really link it to training. It is not long before it starts to become clear that we cannot fulfil the fundamental requirement to be able to state that, 'I am training x because it affects y, which we know is an element of the result'. This is a problem.

Instead we must step away from a generic team view of our physical data and tackle performance enhancement with a more individual approach. This thought process leads us to **'Athletic ability to support specific role requirements'**. This is a key statement which underpins the performance enhancement strategy and is discussed in greater detail in Chapter 9. However, it is crucial to understand that there are two categories of

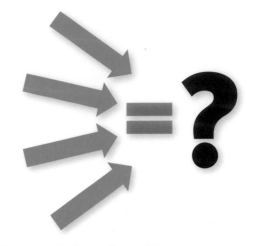

Figure 2.3 The Input–Output Dilemma: we measure everything, but what does it mean?

physical quality which must be addressed. The first is the baseline qualities required by all players to play the game at the requisite level. These factors are constant and can be thought of in terms of a threshold response rather than a dose response (i.e. you just need ENOUGH, rather than 'more is better'). Certain levels of metabolic fitness, speed, agility, etc., are prerequisites for playing at a given level. However, increasing these factors will not necessarily enhance performance. Rather, once these constant general levels of physical ability have been met, the potential for performance enhancement is very dependent on the role of the player. It should be noted that this goes beyond just 'position specific' but is **role specific**. For example, Dimitar Berbatov relies on skill and intelligent movement to gain an advantage without covering much ground. Subsequently, enhancing his aerobic fitness is unlikely to affect his performance. However, in a winger whose game is based on using pace to beat defenders, there is a much stronger case that he will be able to take advantage of power and speed enhancement.

2.2 Underpinning Philosophy

I have had the pleasure of working with some truly excellent S&C coaches during my career. You can read all the books in the world, but there's no substitute for sharing experiences and ideas with another passionate professional day-in, day-out. What is interesting, though, is that even though I have worked side-by-side with these coaches, some of them for years, we still do things very differently. We are all effective and each can stand alone and demonstrate that we have achieved results, but our methods are never identical. This is one of the great things which make S&C so interesting. If there were only one way to do things our programmes would all be the same, our coaching styles would be identical and life would be very dull. Thankfully there is plenty of room for individuality, creativity and an individual philosophy.

The performance model I have described above is non-negotiable in my view. It simply states what matters in football. Coaches may describe it in different ways, but the questions the game asks of us remain the same. How we answer them is a different matter entirely. This is where the coach's philosophy comes into play. What we are about to discuss is a synopsis of how I think best to answer the football question.

My philosophy is based on a system in which the priority of training is based on a hierarchical structure that places primary emphasis on the prevention of injury. This comes from the belief that elite levels of performance will be best achieved through uninterrupted, year-on-year, technical and physical progression. **It is central to the philosophy that this is the way in which S&C can make a more effective contribution to professional football.** I believe the key to this lies in movement mechanics. The best movers get

injured less, simple. Take players like Messi or Ibrahimovic. Both have accumulated a phenomenal number of games at the highest level, generally while being marked men. A major factor in this is their excellent movement patterns. The high-speed, multi-directional demands of football can be incredibly stressful on the body. Inefficient movement and poor distribution of force will multiply this, and injury becomes inevitable. Too often though, the opportunity to improve movement in the gym is ignored in favour of adding load to the bar in search of more strength and power. I think this is short-sighted, though. By

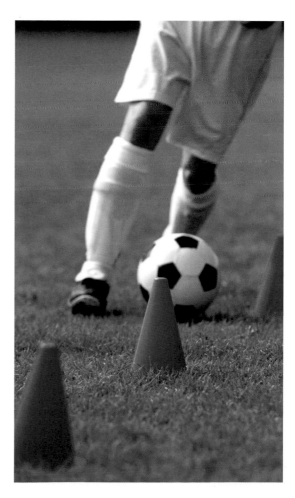

optimising mechanics in fundamental movements, the player has a greater opportunity to express their existing physical qualities more effectively. Therefore there is no trade-off between mechanical optimisation for injury prevention versus performance enhancement, as the same methods provide the quickest route to both.

The schematic in Figure 2.4 below describes the order of progression of training emphasis. It should be noted that initial levels remain constant rather than being replaced by the next. It is also important not to become a slave to the model. Training can be refreshed through mixed modes rather than always programming the perfect technical session.

So, good movement which doesn't place excessive stress on the system is key. But, that takes time to develop. What happens while your players are developing their movement abilities? In the

absence of optimal mechanics, tissue tolerance provides the most reliable way of protecting against strain on the body. Changes in mechanics can often be slow to come to fruition. What's more, the chaotic nature of movement in football, along with the combined effects of fatigue, mean that the tissues will inevitably come under stress regardless of mechanics.

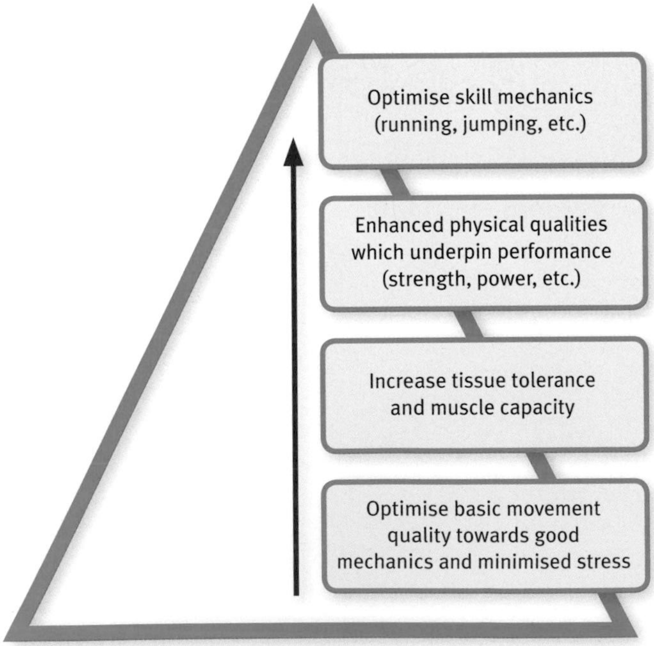

It could be argued that increasing tissue tolerance should be considered the first level of training so that this 'insurance policy' is in place as early as possible. However, whole-body movements designed to affect mechanics (such as squat variations) will also improve tissue tolerance in a more global manner. Therefore it is not a case of either/or.

With regard to direct performance enhancement work I believe that the most effective route is to initially target the strength qualities which underpin running, jumping, cutting, etc. Most players are relatively untrained in these qualities, and so they represent an area with large potential for improvement. Conversely, changes in technique of running, etc., within a game may be hard to effect and produce minimal gains. Perhaps the exception to this is jump mechanics. Developing these in the gym can be important as it leads to more effective expression of force and therefore a greater potential for physical improvement. This work needs to be relevant but not specific. By giving the player the 'raw ingredients' the player has the opportunity to 'turn these into football' during the highly specific challenges faced daily during training. This argument and its physiological basis will be discussed in much more detail in Chapter 10.

Finally, technical changes to movement mechanics can be considered the 'icing on the cake'. It is

Figure 2.4 Priority of Training

Optimise skill mechanics (running, jumping, etc.)

Enhanced physical qualities which underpin performance (strength, power, etc.)

Increase tissue tolerance and muscle capacity

Optimise basic movement quality towards good mechanics and minimised stress

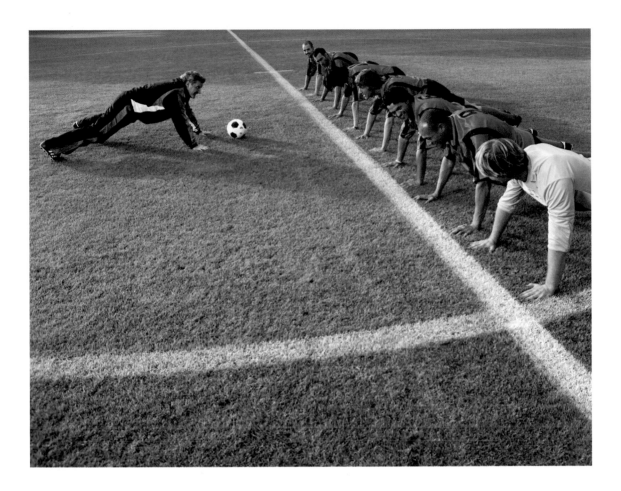

worth giving close consideration to how much time is spent on this area, the potential for change and the impact on performance. It is also important to remember that poor technique may frequently be the result of physical deficit, and so these must be addressed in tandem. In the same vein, technical improvements are likely to have the most success where the player's body is 'taught' how to move properly through coaching manipulations rather than through cognitive learning. It is unrealistic to expect a player to focus on mechanics in play, and therefore they are best served by being given the capacity to perform correctly, which the body will then self-select.

2.3 Summary

In this chapter we have explored the question of exactly how S&C can enhance football performance, or more accurately, how football performance can be enhanced by S&C (if you don't understand the difference, please read this chapter again before progressing). I have described the broad outlines of my own philosophy and how I work to affect these areas. Later we will talk about the specific methods and systems which I have found effective. Before we jump to that though, there is the small matter of how to get your message across in the first place which must be addressed, and the dark art of coaching ...

003
systems of delivery

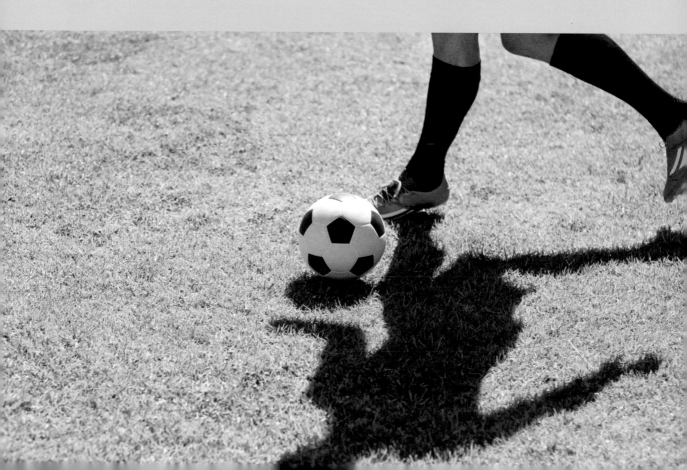

'It's not what you do, it's the way that you do it'. Maybe not the most original or inspirational quotation but there's a lot of truth in it. While few would disagree in principle, I could quite easily fill these pages purely with technical detail of prescription protocols, scientific rationale and exercise options without anyone batting an eyelid. However, we would all have missed one of the most important elements of successful S&C: HOW do you deliver your message?

To some, it may have never occurred that there is another way of doing things. For others, they may have no control of many of these factors. Even if this is the case, it is still worth spending quality time giving consideration to such matters. I have often been left frustrated in conversation with football practitioners who fail to let their imagination travel beyond the constraints imposed upon them from day to day. I frequently found that whenever trying to debate an interesting concept the reply would all too swiftly come back, '... but the problem in football is ...'. You may not be able to change it today or even tomorrow, but if you haven't set your mind free to design your Utopia, how will you ever begin your journey to get there?

In order for the S&C practitioner to justify the title of 'coach' the method of 'teaching' must be given due consideration rather than simply writing programmes regardless of the environment or players involved. Like all sports, football has its own identity in terms of typical personality types and the cultural environment. Consequently, using coaching methods which work in other sports, such as track and field, may not be appropriate in football. There are no correct or incorrect methods. However the S&C coach should be aware of all the choices available and the cost/benefits of each. This will enable more precision, and ultimately success, in coaching. Through this chapter we will explore coaching methods and how we construct sessions to optimise learning.

3.1 Coach:Player Ratios

How many players do you have in a session with you? More interestingly, how did you come about that number? Is that the maximum number before things descend into chaos? Is that just who turns up? Or is that just the capacity of the room you train in? It is worth exploring what our options are and when we might prefer fewer players, and when more is better.

The Group Session

To some extent this may simply come down to available resources, and there is no alternative to group sessions. Aside from efficiency, the group session does offer some advantages. Sessions requiring a high intensity of effort will undoubtedly be greater with the atmosphere and competition of the group (provided it is channelled appropriately). There is also likely to be a greater testosterone response to the session in this environment due to the potential for positive psycho-social hormonal interactions in groups of male players, which can enhance both performance and adaptation. It is important that the S&C coach is well-organised in such a session, to ensure that programming can be tweaked for individual needs, and high-quality coaching interventions can still be delivered effectively through 'controlling the room'. Of course there is an inevitable compromise in coaching detail in such an environment. One simple formula I like to bear in mind in these situations is:

$$\text{Player focus} = \frac{\text{Coach's Voice}}{\text{No. of players}}$$

17

This can potentially lead to changes in programming. If I want a high level of training intensity I am likely to opt for a larger group. However, the coaching and technical side may be compromised, so my exercise selections need to reflect this. That is to say, I will choose options that are less technically demanding (e.g. jump squats rather than Olympic lifts).

The Individual or Small-Numbers Group Session

The individual session certainly offers the opportunity for more bespoke programming and focused coaching. The absence of distraction from other players may also promote greater levels of concentration (and possibly even effort). Therefore, sessions in which QUALITY of movement is more important than QUANTITY of movement are likely to be more effective when the coach:player ratio is at its lowest.

We can actually attempt to get the best of both worlds and create an individual session within a group session. It is easy to hide in a large group and get away with poor technique. By breaking the group into smaller groups the coach does not have to watch everyone at once. This can be extended by unofficially nominating an exercise which you wish to put the most coaching focus on, and directing attention disproportionately to this area.

Table 3.1 below summarises the pros and cons of group versus individual sessions.

3.2 Who to Work With

Elite sport is a cut-throat business. Resources are finite and should always be directed to the point of greatest impact – even when the budget runs to millions. That alone makes the question of who to work with a worthwhile one. While all members of the squad are important, it would be would naïve to suggest that some aren't more important than others. There is also the issue of how much a player can gain from working with you. Are they at a high risk of injury? Are their trainable physical qualities ones which will directly enhance their performance? I would never turn a keen and

Table 3.1	Group vs. Individual Sessions	
	Individual Session	**Group Session**
Pros	Precise coaching and programming	Time-efficient
	Optimal levels of concentration	Intense atmosphere
	Calm environment	Competition among players
	Some players enjoy feeling valued	Good hormonal primer
Cons	Lack of intensity/boredom	Compromised organisation
	Non-compliant players feel 'picked on'	Distracting influences
	Drain on resources	Lack of programming & coaching precision

enthusiastic player away, and of course, everyone has something they can work on which is worth doing. Sometimes though, it is important not to just go to the wheel that is squeaking the loudest. The chances are that the guy who loves the gym and is full of questions will end up drawing you away from others who are less keen. The problem is, he most likely needs you least as he's already working. If he isn't a priority player then you could well be missing a trick. I'm comfortable admitting that I have had mornings where I may have only worked with one player in a session that lasted 15 minutes. I walked out into the car park happy with my contribution though. I knew I had grabbed THE key player that day (due to a combination of injury risk and importance to the team) and, thanks to great communication with the medical department, hit exactly the RIGHT things in those 15 minutes.

Ultimately there tends to be a group within the squad who will suffer the most injury, and the loss of whom will damage the team the most. If these players are targeted and their issues identified, it is possible to be much more strategic, and ultimately impactful. I have seen this approach be highly successful first-hand, and firmly believe that it is completely appropriate to give a lot to a few rather than a little to everyone.

A very simplistic method of determining priority is simply to assign a nominal value to importance in the team and clinical risk/potential for performance gains (depending on the purpose of the training). See table 3.2 for an example.

As you can see, this provides a means of comparing the priority of two players of quite different make-up. It should be noted that both of these qualities are entirely fluid rather than fixed. If the first-choice goalkeeper is struggling with an injury then the importance of the reserve keeper is likely to increase dramatically. Similarly, the clinical picture may change very quickly through the rehab process. Even trainability may reduce as a player starts to plateau and gains drop off.

3.3 Producing a Bespoke System of Delivery

The debate presented so far has been fairly binary: groups or individuals; work with a priority player or not. In reality of course we are not restricted to such rigid thinking. In fact, creative thinking and a tailor-made approach to your own club/squad is essential if your S&C set-up is to be as effective as possible. Throughout my time in football the way in which S&C has been delivered has generally changed to some extent every season. This may be the result of greater or lesser buy-in from a manager, changes in the playing personnel and their needs, changes in S&C staffing, etc. Football is an environment of constant change and so in turn, we need to be able change with it in order to provide an effective service.

Table 3.2	Example nominal values		
	Importance	**Clinical Risk/Trainability**	**Priority**
Player A	8	5	13/20
Player B	4	7	11/20

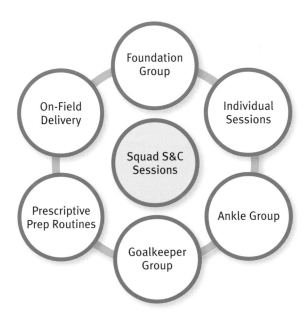

Figure 3.1 Example Delivery Model

The schematic in Figure 3.1 illustrates an example model of delivery which uses a broad strategy to provide a range of options. This caters for compliant and non-compliant players (i.e. combination of mandatory training to provide a minimal dose plus an option of more). Pockets of high-importance players are targeted such as the high-priority development group. Key time-loss injuries are addressed through specific small sessions with players who have been identified as 'at risk' directed towards the sessions. There are an infinite number of other ways to cater to the squad. Ultimately it is about assessing the needs, the resources and taking a creative approach to finding the best solutions.

Gym versus Outdoor Environment

An element of football culture dictates that many pros will consider anything performed on grass as part of their job whereas inside, gym-based work is an extra or a punishment. The same view is sometimes taken by coaches and managers. Consequently, whole-squad buy-in can sometimes be easier to achieve outside than in. Pitch-based work can also be more time-efficient and appear more integrated with the coaching staff, with whom it is easier to engage in dialogue around what you are trying to achieve.

Ultimately though, the pitch was designed for playing football and the gym was designed for strength and conditioning, and so the latter will always be more suitable for developing raw physical qualities within the first three elements of our pyramid of priorities in Chapter 2 (fundamental movement ability, tissue tolerance and underpinning physical qualities). There may be various reasons for having to conduct all physical preparation outside, many of which may be out of the S&C coach's control. I firmly believe, though, that if the choice is available the gym should be used where possible as it allows us to 'give them what they don't get on the pitch'.

Of course, the outdoor environment is best suited to level 4 of the coaching system (specific skill performance). However, it is critical that this is done with high quality. Therefore the coach must be careful to ensure that the group dynamic is correct. We know that player focus can often be poor in large groups, and a technical movement session (which relies on focus and attention by the player) can end up being worthless. A good example of this can often be seen when attempting to work on running mechanics in large groups. Of course, one where intensity is key (such as sprints) will benefit from this (see above). There are methods available to increase technical quality, even in a group setting – which leads us on to the art of coaching by stealth.

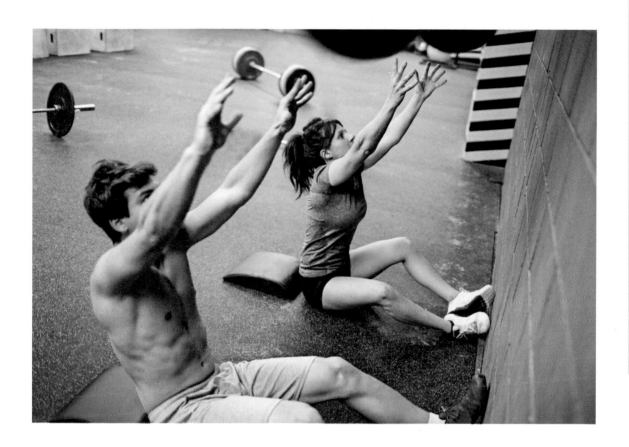

Coaching by Stealth

One of the most important lessons I learnt after
moving from track and field back into football was
that the differences between these two creatures
were much more than simply their physical
attributes. Many who chose athletics could also
have been successful in football and vice-versa.
The reasons behind this are of course myriad.
However, a key factor lies in what makes them
'tick'. For example, do you enjoy functioning as
part of a team, or are you more individually
focused? Do you enjoy the challenge of focusing
on one particular skill and perfecting it, or do you
thrive off the chaos and rapid stimulus provided by
an interactive team sport? These have big
implications on how best to motivate a person,
how they learn and how to coach them.

Football players are often not accustomed to high
levels of concentration, technical focus and intense
effort during non-footballing activities. This is
often evident in the warm-up, where players who
have achieved high levels of technical excellence
in football skills are seen performing simple
dynamic flexibility exercises with poor focus and
technique.

In my view it is a common mistake born of a lack of
understanding and lazy thinking to take training
methods from one world and transpose them
wholesale into another, assuming they will
automatically work in the same way. Let me give
you an example. Track and field athletes use
hurdle walk-though drills to achieve a number of
goals including hip mobility, trunk control,

coordination, etc. These are all qualities which you would want to see in a footballer, so surely it makes sense to incorporate them into your practice? Well maybe, but we need to think about some key considerations. The essence of these drills is that the value comes from performing them as close to perfection as possible. If great focus isn't given to postural control then the trunk transfer is lost. If form is not maintained and elements of 'cheating' come in, then the hips won't be taken into the ranges required to develop mobility. Worst of all, poor form has the potential to see the player rehearsing dysfunctional movement patterns and ingraining issues we are

trying to address. I saw this issue first hand when I was once asked to run some ad hoc hurdle work with players as part of a warm-up. By setting the practice up in a way which requires the players to focus diligently on form, I was never going to get the high level of application in each and every player that I needed to see.

Of course, this issue isn't limited to transferring from athletics. I tend to think that S&C coaches are the magpies of sports science. We steal our methods from all kinds of environment, all with their own distinct idiosyncrasies. Olympic lifts can be a great tool. Remember though, weightlifters

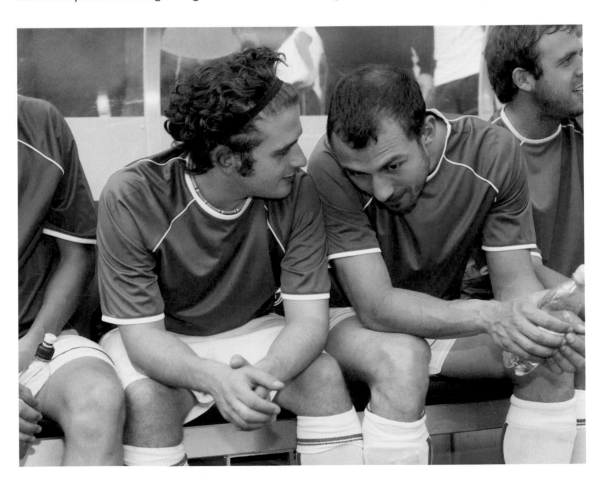

have spent years honing the ability to summon all of their explosive abilities in an instant – not all players demonstrate this in the gym. I could cite 100 similar examples, as I'm sure you could. It simply underlines the message that what you do counts, but so does the way that you do it.

It is all too easy to continue prescribing exercises in this manner and simply blame the players for their poor focus. However, this is to ignore the obvious and accept failure. The coach must either change the behaviour of the players, or adapt exercises so that the technical error is removed and good technique is inevitable. I call this **coaching by stealth**. In the hurdle example above I quickly realised that the players weren't really at fault. In their minds they were giving an appropriate level of concentration. Unlike a sprinter though, this feels very peripheral to them and it is unrealistic to expect them to apply the same level of application as you would hope to see when perfecting a football skill. At this point I was faced with a critical choice. Option 1 was to blame the players and join the ranks of defeated practitioners who spend their time criticising players. Option 2 was to recognise that my methods weren't working, and adapt them. In this example I adapted the drill slightly in ways which meant the technical errors I was seeing were automatically eradicated (such as pausing above the hurdle to stop the use of momentum and keeping a ball above the head to address posture). Now all of a sudden we had tweaked the methods and 100% of the players were making the shapes I needed to see, regardless of their level of motivation or interest. In an ideal world we would educate the players as to the value of all the work we prescribe and they would treat it with the same level of focus as football training. In reality though, this requires a lot of work and will never be 100% foolproof. That certainly doesn't mean that we give

up on the aspiration, we just need something else to guarantee the quality of our work in the meantime.

Positive Pollution

To be considered fully effective, a coach should have scale to their work. By that I mean that they have the ability to create influence and impact broadly and not just limited to the players with whom they work directly. One of the most gratifying sights to me was walking into the gym and seeing a player I had never coached performing exercises or techniques I knew I had brought to the club.

Anyone who has ever been in a gym at a football club will know that players performing their own self-directed work do not generally wander in with a clear routine and protocol. Exercise selection tends to be very reactive, i.e. what equipment is out and who is doing what. Often they will perform the exercises that they know and are comfortable with, for these reasons alone rather than a targeted outcome. It is also common to see players work on pieces of equipment which are set up and available to them (e.g. bench press). Therefore if we change the gym set-up we can change habits, and by exposing players to good practice we can often make their repertoire of familiar exercises more appropriate.

Even before the first coffee of the day I would always head to the gym to make sure that the squat stands had not been dropped down to make a bench press (and quickly remedy it if they had). Over time I removed the option to do this at all and set up a comprehensive suspension training area. Crucially I then worked with a couple of the gym's most 'regular clients' to show them some suitable challenges. I then just had to sit back and let the influence spread. Sure enough, the prison-style bench press club quickly disbanded!

Similarly, it is rare to find a player whose gym routine doesn't include some element of trunk work (generally referred to by players as 'core' but it is often clear the focus is abs). Again the choice of exercise often comes from friends, magazines, etc. By simply exposing players to more suitable alternatives which will achieve both function and aesthetics (rather than just the latter), it is possible to keep all parties happy.

3.4 Minimal Dose Philosophy

There are a number of sports in which the question around training volume focuses on a philosophy of 'more is better' or 'how strong can I get'. I would argue that the opposite view should be taken in football though. There are so many different elements that can comprise a training regime, and so many aspects of a player's game to work on, that each element must truly justify its place at the table. Availability of both time and energy of players in the gym will always exist in competition with the demands of playing and training. Therefore we need to be confident that every ounce of energy and every minute in the gym could not have been spent more productively elsewhere. This means making our programmes as lean as possible and achieving the desired effect with maximum efficiency.

This leads us to the minimum dose philosophy of training. Good evidence has been presented to demonstrate that by maintaining a high intensity of training it is possible to maintain gains with very low volumes of work. This may mean dropping the volume of work required to achieve gains to as little as 40% for maintenance. This is critical with the rehabbing player, as willingness to perform

gym work almost always reduces following return to training and playing. Interestingly, it has also been shown that one session per week is sufficient to maintain gains (e.g. pre-season gains) whereas once per fortnight is not. This vindicates the practice of a once-per-week squad session and suggests that there may be efficacy in this approach.

I have applied these principles in mini case study examples on a number of occasions and found them to be highly effective. Not only were strength gains maintained but the practice of aiming for a minimal dose also achieved a much greater adherence rate to sessions after returning to training from injury. This is very much a case of being able to achieve 100% of a low-volume goal rather than 0% of a more ambitious programme.

3.5 Communicating the Message

We've already seen countless examples of the importance of the way in which training is delivered. However, there are also more subtle elements of communication in terms of how your message is conveyed. This comes down to professional relationships. There are a few simple rules which underpin good practice. In some ways these should be obvious and not worth stating. However, I know from having seen them broken countless times that this message needs to be repeated.

The first is to realise that the players are not your friends. These lines can get blurred sometimes due to the informal nature of the gym and the frequency of contact. However, it is important to draw a line. Becoming excessively close with a player will compromise your professional boundaries. Alongside this comes the reminder that your role to them is as a person whose knowledge and advice they respect and trust. They do not need a new best friend. Consequently, dressing like a player (including hair-cuts, jewellery and tattoos), and attempting to lead and discuss a football-like lifestyle is a backward step. You are much more use to them if they think you spend your evenings at home buried in books or training yourself, rather than being out doing a poor impersonation of a player.

Another important rule is the old cliché of under-promise and over-deliver. It dawned on me relatively early on in my career just how many people end up promising to make huge gains to a top player's performance. Imagine a typical player who may have gone through an Academy and then gone on to play for maybe three or four clubs through their professional career. Even without staff turnover that's a whole lot of physios,

coaches, nutritionists and sports scientists all telling the player how much they can help them. That's before we've even considered the sales reps, glory hunters and well-meaning friends who all have advice. Given that the player has already had a good measure of success they are right to be sceptical when scores of people all think they can add 50% to their game. So with all that in the background, I realised that joining the long queue of people promising the Earth was unlikely to create much inspiration. Along the same lines, players also do not enjoy long anatomy and physiology lectures that give great detail and show how knowledgeable you are. However, players do generally have a good sense of whether an exercise is going to work for them.

So in my view, say little, show them something very good and let the quality of your work sell itself.

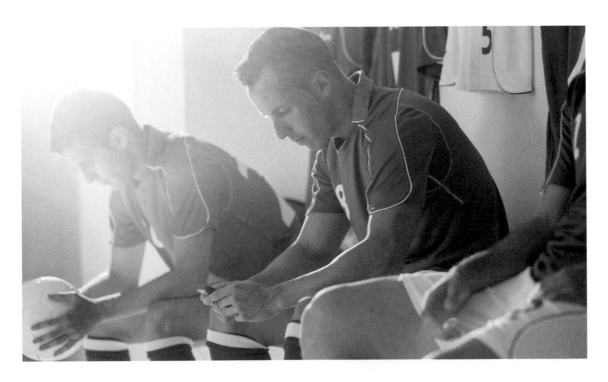

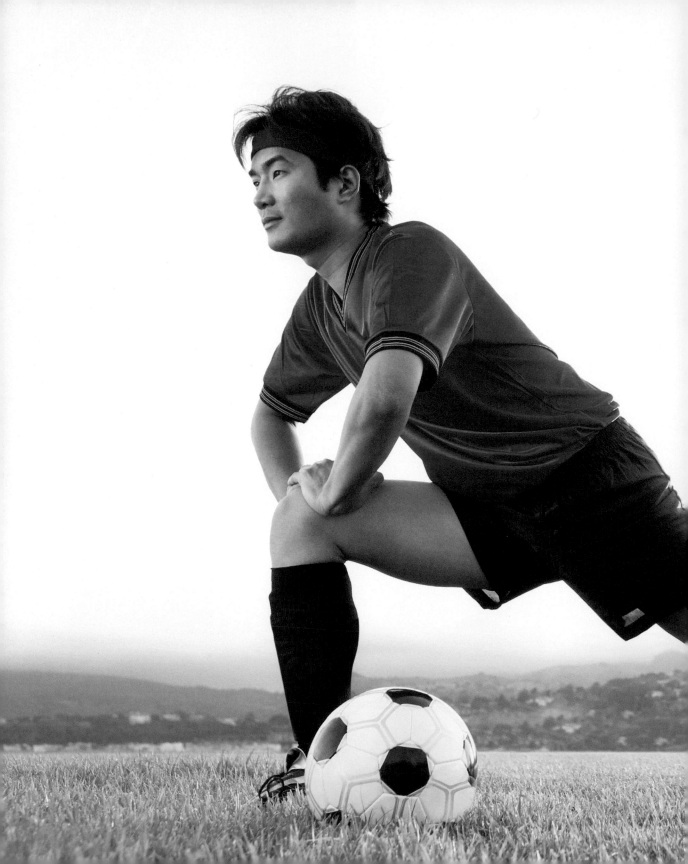

part 2

injury
prevention

004
model of injury prevention

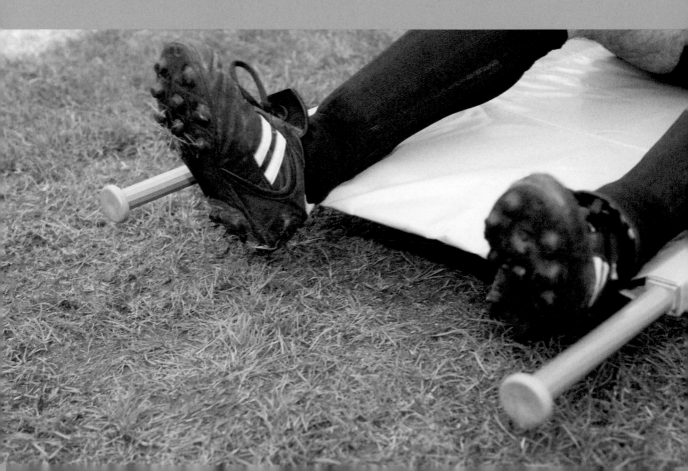

The first goal of any S&C programme should always be injury prevention. Some level of injury is the only guarantee in any sporting career. However, the risk of injury, the frequency, the severity, and the time to recover from injury can all be reduced.

Injury can be incredibly destructive. The journey of top-level performers to the pinnacle of their trade is completed in small, gradual steps. Every injury sets this journey back. It is not just the time taken to return to training which should be counted, but also the return to the previous level of performance. It is not until this point is reached that the developmental journey can be resumed. When these lost opportunities are accumulated they can add up to a sizeable proportion of a player's short career. Furthermore, the attrition which is suffered by the body can start to set back a player's physical potential. We have seen many times the player formerly full of pace who has been slowed by countless hamstring injuries and tissue scarring. Similarly, osteochondral defects can be hugely destructive to the point of restricting the ability to achieve some of the fundamental movement patterns which underpin performance.

If this paints a depressing picture of injury, it shouldn't. What I am attempting to do is illustrate the scale of the opportunity we have in front of us. If anything, this picture should excite you as it leads us to the realisation that we can really add significant value to the player, the squad and the football club.

4.1 Injury Prevention – Beyond Prehab

If we are to have any chance of affecting injuries we first need to understand the true nature of the problem. If we take a narrow-minded view of the problem it is easy to run swiftly to the safety of our coaching toolbox and start planning exercises and training regimes. However, to be effective we need to treat the problem as well as the symptoms.

Football training and games cause close to 100% of injuries. Or to put it another way, *excessive* football causes injuries. This may be due to the total volume of work, an overload of one specific element of work due to the shape of training, etc. This inescapable truth somehow seems to elude many overseers in football. Managers will often talk of how they have had 'horrendous luck with injuries'. In other sports, coaches whose athletes are regularly injured will soon suffer tarnished reputations. In football this connection is often not made though. Instead it is much more common for an external audit of the medical department to be commissioned!

My point here is not to instigate a blame game of medical versus coaching departments, this happens far too much already. Instead I merely wish to encourage S&C practitioners to take a global view of the problem. After all, if we are to be held accountable for our ability to minimise injury isn't it only fair that we have some say over the key variables? Figure 4.1 below illustrates the counterbalanced relationship between training

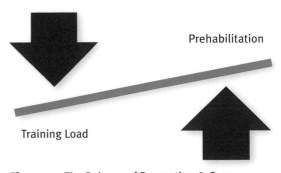

Figure 4.1 The Balance of Prevention & Cure

load and preventative work. While risk can undoubtedly be offset by prehabilitation interventions, the risk is never removed entirely, and every player will have a training threshold beyond which they will break.

If it is not already clear that, as S&C coaches, we do not have 100% ownership of the injury prevention problem, Figure 4.2 illustrates all of the key stakeholders. Consequently, as a team we must be able to coordinate, analyse, predict and be proactive. Of course this will not all fall on the shoulders of the S&C coach. However, the savvy practitioner will quickly realise that building effective relationships will have a huge influence on how impactful their work will be. This is an

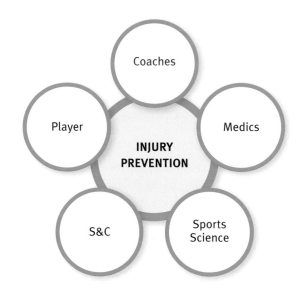

Figure 4.2 Stakeholders in Player Health

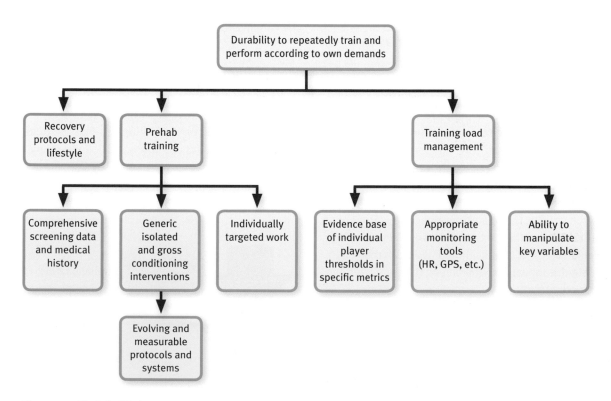

Figure 4.3 Model of Robustness

example of a situation where leadership is required regardless of job title or status.

This view of injury prevention in the broader context is captured in the model of robustness in Figure 4.3.

4.2 A Model of Injury Prevention

Having established that a fully effective injury prevention model should include a significant focus on intelligent management of training load, we can now turn our attention to the other side of the coin in direct delivery of exercise to reduce risk.

In simplistic terms, non-contact injury occurs when the mechanical stress tolerance of a tissue is exceeded. This can be acute as the result of a sudden catastrophic force overload, such as landing awkwardly. Alternatively the issue may be chronic through an accumulated stress over time when tissues have not healed from micro-trauma between stresses (i.e. overuse injury). We therefore have two potential routes to reducing injury: reducing the likelihood or extent to which tissues are being overloaded; and/or increasing the capacity of the tissues to tolerate load.

Reducing the Mechanical Burden

We may wish to reduce the risk of an acute injury through a single violent episode such as a fall or collision. Of course we cannot prevent injury through direct trauma. However, we can equip a player to be able to resist soft tissue injuries that result from the body being forced into unnatural positions, such as those often seen during ACL (anterior cruciate ligament) ruptures. The disproportionate stress placed on the vulnerable structures is likely to far exceed their natural tolerance. Therefore attempts to increase the

A Question of Strength

The learned coach, scientist and motor learning guru Frans Bosch would argue that '...strength does not exist as an isolated quality'. By regarding strength purely as a motor property it is not possible to separate the two component parts of the term neuro-muscular. To some extent I agree. However, through our injury-prevention model we will need to break this rule. My defence of this approach comes from the fact that we may employ neural-control techniques which are low intensity and do not affect the structure of the musculature involved. Conversely, we seek to improve tissue tolerance and force production through methods which bear little resemblance to the functional motor requirements of a task, but target protein synthesis and increases in muscle-tissue quality and quantity.

Of course, these qualities are far from mutually exclusive, and where possible we should seek to train them in unison. We just don't need to be a slave to such constraints. Therefore we can legitimately discuss methods which target neural control, muscular capacity or neuromuscular strength.

tolerance of these tissues to the point whereby they can withstand such an episode are unlikely to be successful. Instead we may wish to focus on developing neuromuscular strength, so that the player has an enhanced ability to maintain optimal posture and positions. This is important as it supports the use of high force, whole-body exercises as part of our injury-prevention strategy. It may surprise many that studies of the effectiveness of exercise in reducing injury have found strength to be the single most important quality.

The mechanism of injury described above is based upon large forces which take a player dramatically outside of their normal patterns of movement. Conversely, chronic injury tends to occur from the accumulated stress sustained within *normal movement patterns*. All training will involve placing stress on tissues, but provided sufficient recovery for repair between bouts is allowed (through rest, nutrition, etc.), this will not result in injury. If the volume of stress exceeds the ability to recover, then injury will eventually occur. However, the degree of stress sustained during a given workload can be exacerbated by movement dysfunctions. Therefore by correcting dysfunction, the trauma associated with a given workload can be reduced and the player's capacity to train without injury is increased. Once again, this may be addressed through enhancing neuromuscular strength. There are several other mechanisms which also come to the fore. Neuromuscular control is certainly key for correcting dysfunction, both in terms of achieving sufficient activation of the relevant musculature and the ability of the nervous system to produce an appropriately coordinated response to achieve the desired movement (or non-movement) outcome. Movement dysfunction is also affected by structural issues such as range of movement (ROM) and tissue length. It should be noted that tissue length may refer to muscle, tendon, ligament, neural tissue and myofascia. It is also possible that laxity may cause a dysfunction rather than simply tightness. The 'quality' of tissue is also important. Athletes may often complain of feeling tight despite no changes in ROM.

Increasing Tissue Tolerance

The capacity of the tissues to tolerate stress may come via greater structural integrity, greater ability to produce force, or greater resistance to fatigue. After performing conditioning-type exercise there follows an increase in collagen synthesis in both tendon and muscle tissue. This adds to the tensile strength of the tissues and their capacity to resist deformation. Importantly this adds to both the size (cross-sectional area) and quality (mechanical stiffness) of the tendon. A reduction in neovascularisation (a proliferation of blood vessels into a tendon causing pain) is also a key outcome from loading the patella tendon.

Hopefully it is not necessary in a text of this nature to list the various adaptations which occur within a muscle to enhance force production. If the strength of a vulnerable muscle group is increased, then the risk of an injury resulting from high-intensity actions is reduced. An obvious example of this can be found in the hamstrings: by increasing the eccentric strength of this muscle group to a point whereby they can match the concentric force of the opposing muscle group.

Similarly, in addition to increasing a muscle's capacity to produce force, it is also desirable to minimise the loss of force production potential to fatigue. Raising the metabolic capacity of a muscle through increases in mitochondria, increased capillarisation, etc., may subsequently help to preserve force production throughout matches and training. In should also be noted that further to these local adaptations, central metabolic fitness is also fundamental in this role and highlights the importance of the on-field conditioner (among others) in contributing to this goal.

In summary, our ability to directly reduce the risk of injury comes through a combination of reducing the mechanical stress suffered by the player and increasing their capacity to tolerate such stress. This is summarised in Figure 4.4 below.

The Tools of Risk Reduction

Our journey into injury prevention thus far has taken a 'top-down' approach. By this I mean that we have started by evaluating the issue globally and identifying exactly how much of the problem we actually own. Having done that we have now been clear in describing the mechanisms by which our exercise interventions may reduce risk. Only now is it appropriate for us to start discussing specific methodologies and protocols. I hope that the discussion so far has made it clear why such an approach is so important. We now have assurance that our work will be impactful but also understand its limitations and the bigger picture. This is very different to the traditional 'solution first' thinking where we begin with some exercises and work upwards.

Part of the value of being very clear and precise in terms of the adaptations we are seeking to achieve is that programming becomes very easy. It also provides us with the freedom and licence to put our own stamp on our programmes. This moves us away from pointless arguments such as high force versus functional trainers. Instead we are able to critically evaluate our work by reviewing whether or not the desired adaptations occurred, and what impact this had on injury incidence. We will discuss the various key methodologies in the coming pages. Every coach will have their own bias and preferred methods. Some will love the barbell, while others swear by yoga. I will give you my own views on what I have found to be most effective and how to get the best from each. However, provided you are able to clearly articulate what you are trying to achieve and understand the

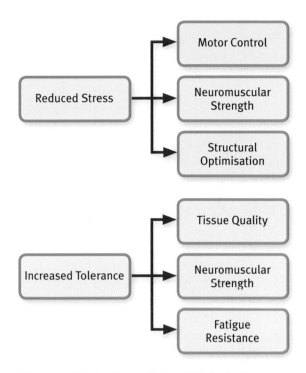

Figure 4.4 Mechanisms of Injury Risk Reduction

exercise tools you use, then you are free in the knowledge that there are many routes to Rome.

4.3 Barbell Exercises

If we refer back to Figure 2.4 in Chapter 2, the foundation of the training priority pyramid is 'Optimise basic movement quality towards good mechanics and minimised stress'. This is placed ahead of 'Increase tissue tolerance and muscle capacity'. As has already been mentioned, the latter of these can arguably be achieved more quickly than the former. On that basis it may seem logical to work on the quickest win first. The reason that I do not take that approach is that barbell exercises can be used to improve both movement quality and tissue tolerance, without having to make a choice between one and the other.

In my view, barbell exercises are fabulously effective and terribly misunderstood in equal measure. If we refer back to Figure 4.4 (Mechanisms of Injury Risk Reduction), barbell exercises have the capacity to impact on all six aspects of risk reduction. Neuromuscular control is challenged through the need to maintain posture against the overload of the bar, and through challenging mechanics such as unilateral or overhead lifts. While increased neuromuscular strength may be obvious, structural optimisation may be less so. However, the opportunity to regain the natural 'normal' mobility and range around the hips and ankles via barbell lifts should not be overlooked. Furthermore, the weight room, in contrast to the football pitch, naturally produces high levels of mechanical impulse with low impact. This is ideal for improving tissue quality as it results in high protein synthesis with low protein degradation.

However, that is not to say that simply turning up and doing some squats will do the job. The precision in programming, coaching and performing these movements is absolutely paramount to their efficacy. My approach has long been that these movements are primarily opportunities to improve the QUALITY of a player's movement rather than the QUANTITY. With this in mind, the range and control of movement become much more important than the load. I'm sure most would agree with me on this in principle. However, it is amazing how often I see this rule contradicted. Maybe not to gross extremes, but very often a few extra kilos are added and range is reduced slightly, or control is not quite optimal. For me, the load on the bar simply needs to be sufficient to promote an adaptation, be that to neural control or to find new ROM in tight structures. As a result I am very comfortable working with low–moderate loads of

A Word on Squats

I have often said that I can solve any movement question as long as the answer is squats. Although this may not quite be true there is much to be said for the sacred squat. Tight ankles are ubiquitous in football, and not only carry increased risk locally, but also affect movement in other areas such as hip extension in running. There is no doubt in my mind that squats are more effective than any combination of isolated exercises and massage treatments in improving ankle ROM.

If we move on to the glutes: a good, deep squat not only requires the glutes to work, but critically they do so in a coordinated manner in a functional movement. Therefore for me they have much more value than 'glute exercises' performed in isolation on the floor.

Lastly, the position of the bar in a back squat demands that the player maintain good thoracic posture through extension. The only exception to this is if a 'sissy pad' is used. It is for that very good reason that in my view no football club should own one.

These are just a few of the many benefits of squats to a player. For a deeper discussion I would recommend *Starting Strength* by Mark Ripptoe and *Becoming a Supple Leopard* by Kelly Starrett.

20–50kg (depending on the player and the exercise). Given the nature of the adaptation I am seeking, it seems only logical to base my progressions and overload on greater range or more challenging mechanics.

I have already mentioned that barbell exercises are often misunderstood. To those who do not have an intimate understanding, they are one-dimensional. They are perceived as being a blunt instrument, high intensity in nature and used to increase strength. We have already seen that in the hands of a skilled practitioner they can be so much more. As the S&C coach it is vital that you work hand-in-glove with the medical team, and sometimes coaches and players, to make sure that you do not fall victim to this misunderstanding. All too often an entirely appropriate element of your programme may be withdrawn if others become concerned that the player is 'not ready yet'. When we consider that even light jogging results in forces around twice body weight being tolerated, then the loadings involved in squats, deadlifts and single exercises are minute.

The whole-body nature of these exercises means that they carry the added value of affording the coach an opportunity to assess movement competency. Depending on your point-of-view and access to the player, this can remove the need for formal movement screening. By having these frequent and regular opportunities to assess movement, a greater handle can be gained over how a player is coping with load and adapting to interventions.

The true value of a barbell programme comes from the skill of the coach to match the exercise choice to the requirements of the player and their specific needs and body dimensions. It is then important to be able to make small adjustments to tailor the exercise to the player and their goal, rather than slavishly working towards a rigid technical model of the exercise. As a result, several players may all be doing the same exercise on paper, but the individual tweaks made by the coach will mean that the shapes which they are making have small but critical differences. This is especially true in football, where a player may be 6'6" or 5'2".

4.4 Isolation Exercises

If I were able to use only one type of exercise, it would be those described in the previous section. Thankfully we do not work under such constraints and so it is only logical to use a careful blend of whole-body and isolation exercises.

Again, the value of this tool like any other comes from a clear understanding of the adaptation sought. Let's start with perhaps the most simplistic of all, **increasing the strength of a specific muscle group**. There are circumstances whereby a particular muscle group becomes weak and/or atrophied, perhaps following injury or as a result of movement dysfunction. In such a scenario the musculature in question does not contribute to gross movements in the way in which we would like. This is problematic as continuing to rehearse these movements simply serves to ingrain an unwanted pattern, and fails to elicit the increases in strength in the affected area which we require. Therefore isolated work allows us to target the affected area before it can be 'reintroduced' to the gross pattern. It should be noted that a change in patterning following an isolated intervention is by no means an automatic process, although it is far too often presumed to be so. However, if the issue is that the muscle is simply too small and weak, as opposed to issues around firing and coordination, then it is certainly likely to be an easier task.

In simplistic terms, we can increase the strength of a muscle purely by adding to the quantity of tissue, i.e. an increased cross-sectional area. In the case of atrophied tissue this alone may be enough. If this is the underpinning philosophy being pursued then programming should reflect the goal of hypertrophy accordingly, along with considerations around nutrition and recovery. Of course the chances of successful integration into performance as well as being able to contribute positively to the task should be sought through specificity of the exercise use. One of the key criteria for specificity described by Bosch is, *'The types of muscle action must be similar to those used during competition (intra- and inter- muscular)'* . This requires an understanding of how the musculature functions during the common tasks of play. Of course this may not be a singular choice in either the exercise or the performance task in play. However, the point at which injury is most likely to occur may be identified. The complex nature of the bi-articular hamstring group provides a good example of this. The goal of muscle action specificity should certainly not be confused with attempting to recreate the sports action itself. Ironically, in doing so it is often the case that while joint mechanics may appear similar, the patterns of firing and muscle-tendon unit length changes may be drastically different.

Just as we can add raw material to a muscle group which is found wanting, the same is true of tendons. Both the Achilles and patella tendons are frequent areas of concern for footballers. It is common practice for jumpers in track and field to include isolated tendon-loading exercises as a perennial element of their conditioning programmes, due to the high stress placed on these areas during jumping. Given the prevalence of these injuries in football it would seem sensible to do the same. We have already learnt that tendon quality can be enhanced through appropriate loading strategies. Exercises such as leg extensions and heel raises can be used to load the patella and Achilles tendons respectively. As tendons are not composed of contractile tissue, the time under tension (TUT) becomes of

paramount importance during programming, rather than repetition counting. Much is often made of the value of eccentric training methodologies to target tendon adaptation. However, this has led to some confusion and questionable practice. The eccentric phase of a movement can be used to our advantage as it allows for greater mechanical loading of the tendon (please consult the force–velocity curve if you don't know why). However, this only comes into effect if we use loads that take advantage of this fact. It is common to see players performing eccentrics with loads they can easily move concentrically. This comes from the mistaken belief that there is something intrinsically special about the eccentric phase, which is not true. Isometric training has also been shown to be highly effective in improving the mechanical properties of tendons. This can be particularly useful when working with players who do not tolerate impact well, as this tool can serve as an effective replacement for plyometric work with regard to local adaptation of the tendons.

My colleague and friend Ben Rosenblatt, formerly Lead Rehab Scientist at the British Olympic Intensive Rehab Unit, works on the basis that the collagen synthesis cycle lasts approximately 48 hours. Therefore this appears to be a logical time course for doses of tendon-specific isolated work.

Isolation exercises may also be used to focus on the specifically neural element of neuromuscular strength. Such exercises are often classified as 'remedial' and are most commonly, although certainly not exclusively, used by physios. The goal of this type of intervention is to increase the neural drive to a muscle which is perceived to be underactive. This is likely to be achieved through an increase in motor unit firing rate and synchronisation. This underactivity may be in a

Exposing Our Achilles Heel

It is rare that football teams look across the pond to NFL teams for training lessons, but a valuable one may have been afforded us in the 2011 NFL season. During the pre-season there was a 'lock out' as a result of industrial action by backroom staff. This resulted in a very short pre-season and, in turn, an unprecedented number of Achilles ruptures. Typically the league would see around five ruptures per season. On this occasion there were twelve within the first 2½ weeks of training.

Of course we can only speculate as to the physiological reasons behind this, and clearly the need to rapidly increase training can be labelled as the cause. What this strongly suggests though is that the slower adaptation rates of tendons and the cessation of activity during the summer places tendons in a vulnerable state. This ties in with my own experience of players with tendon issues who often feel worse after several days' rest.

So what is the lesson here? For me this points to a shift in emphasis for off-season programmes. Typically players are given regimes to go away with that maintain body composition, cardiovascular fitness and muscular endurance. However, perhaps we've missed a trick and maintenance of tendon loading should be our priority? Issues of this type in the early weeks of pre-season are often blamed on hard pitches and increases in running volume. Of course these don't help, but maybe we can prepare our players' tendons to cope in a much more effective way?

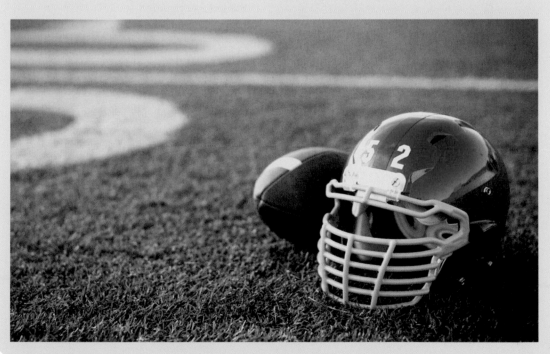

Glutes – Turn On or Turn Off?

It is now highly commonplace to see sports science staff working with players before training or matches performing so-called glute-activation exercises. There are a number of reasons why someone would wish to optimise glute function during performance due to the critical role in actions such as hip extension and knee stability. If you were to ask why these exercises were being performed at this time you would likely receive a response along the lines of, 'I'm *switching on* his glutes'. Such comments are dropped casually into conversation as if the outcome was as sure as night following day. This view is based purely on an assumption that this will have an impact on the neural drive to the glutes during running, etc. More importantly it is one without any solid scientific evidence to back it up. You might ask, 'Where's the harm? Surely it can't hurt so we may as well do it just in case it works?' Well, at best that is highly unscientific. There exists a real possibility that you are wasting valuable preparation time. It may even be possible that you are inducing fatigue in the muscle group and will reduce neural drive in play!

My point is not that this type of work should not be performed. It is simply that to assess the effects in a scientific way and determine the efficacy would not be that difficult. If this is something you believe in and you consider yourself to be based in science, then let's test the hypothesis.

particular movement pattern, such as the activation of the posterior chain during hip extension. Alternatively, there may be a view that a muscle is generally underactive in most common movement patterns. The negative consequence of this is that the force deficit must be compensated for by another muscle group, which subsequently becomes potentially overburdened and vulnerable. Perhaps the most common, and poorly understood, example comes from the glutes and hamstrings.

Exercises designed to target these gains typically use single-joint, slow movements which are closely coached with technique designed to ensure that the targeted musculature is activated. A strong body of evidence exists to support the use of these techniques in making the neural adaptations described. However, once these adaptations have been achieved an alternative paradigm must be pursued. Lederman has described how the specificity of neural patterns in gross movements means that simply 'teaching' a muscle to work does not translate to its automatic incorporation into functional tasks. It is for this reason that such exercises are appropriately considered remedial, and are typically best placed at suitable time points in rehabilitation protocols.

4.5 Plyometrics

If we can agree that our isolated activation exercises are remedial, then we clearly need a method of advancing them, and changing the patterns of muscular activity in gross movements is our end goal. Plyometric exercises are ideally suited to this challenge as they represent a controllable method of producing similar neuromuscular challenges to those seen in game-play tasks. By this I am referring to the greater reliance on elastic strength and reactivity

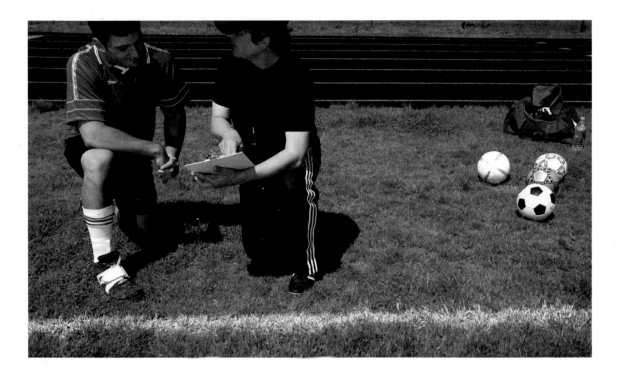

compared with gym exercises. This demands complex neuromuscular skill execution as there is a requirement for pre-activation prior to ground contact, eccentric strength and muscle-tendon stiffness. Rather than motor-unit recruitment being the primary source of adaptation as is seen in isolated work, here the gains are likely to come from inter-muscular coordination and skill development.

Naturally, the type of plyometric exercise that should be used is inherently low level. Far too often this type of work is not given due attention, and progression is made too quickly. Because these exercises are dynamic in their nature they demand a sharp coaching eye to pick up subtle deficiencies in technique. I cannot over-stress the need for the coach to demand precision and excellence in these movements. Because the intensity is naturally low it is imperative that the

focus on skilled execution is high in order for the exercise to carry any value. For this reason I would suggest a very low player:coach ratio. There is always a risk that a player may quickly become bored with this work and so their focus drops and with it so does the level of application and skill. This can be curtailed by effective programming to subtly manipulate the exercise around a theme and so the movement challenge is similar but the player is given variety. This will also aid transfer as a more varied range of skill challenges will assist transfer and retention rather than them simply becoming highly effective within a narrow range. Finally, a great deal of thought should be given to the *type* of coaching cue used. It is widely accepted that cues based on an external focus (directed at the movement effect) are more effective than those promoting an internal focus (directed at the performer's body movements). In other words, they should think about what they need to feel rather than what you as the coach need to see. The ability of a coach to translate this is a critical element of the coaching process which often distinguishes the novice from the expert.

4.6 Yoga

Yoga has had some very good press in football in recent years, principally through the claim that the prolonged career of Ryan Giggs can be attributed to his practice. The presence of yoga in football is far from a new phenomenon though.

Personally I am a big advocate of yoga as an S&C tool. While there are many benefits to yoga, it is most commonly used as a flexibility and mobility aid. If we consider the progress, or lack of it, in our flexibility methods over the last 20 or 30 years it is not surprising that yoga brings something extra. For far too long, our stretching protocols have been based on passive stretches in isolated muscle groups in single planes of movement. Years ago the same could be said of many strength-training methods. Now of course it would be unthinkable to allow such methods to dominate. In the modern era, multi-joint, 'functional' stretches often feature in dynamic warm-ups. However, these tend to serve only as preparation as opposed to developmental work.

In contrast to traditional stretches, yoga poses work through multi-joint challenges and effectively targets myofascial slings which interlink the body. Furthermore, while some elements of passive stretching are a feature, many poses utilise an active stretch which has the added advantage of reciprocal inhibition. The majority of stretching protocols in football carry a very heavy bias towards the lower body. However this often fails to consider the knock-on effect to whole-body

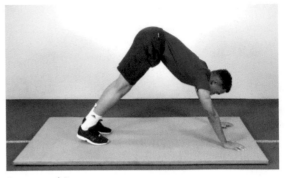

Downward Dog

posture and particularly the impact on gait mechanics. A good example of this can be seen in the implications of poor thoracic posture on the rest of the posterior chain, and the hamstrings in particular. Yoga poses are highly effective tools for altering upper-body posture through strengthening and lengthening appropriately.

If we take the example of the Downward Dog pose we can see from the image above, how a number of factors contribute to developing flexibility through the posterior chain in the areas where we are likely to seek it (i.e. the hamstrings) while retaining posture in areas which require stability such as the lumbar spine.

Of course, we should not fall into the trap of taking a narrow view of yoga as simply a fancy stretch. The capacity to improve posture and control is considerable. Personally I have found yoga to be by far the most effective tool in this area. Considering the importance of posture on mechanics, this is pretty significant. The nature of the poses is such that muscles and connective tissues are lengthened and strengthened in parallel. Furthermore, the requirement to hold poses for extended durations strongly promotes the use of the appropriate level of musculature and avoids compensations. By this I mean that it requires incredible effort to hold a pose using superficial muscles that are intended to function as prime movers. Therefore the player must find an alternative strategy and begin to engage deep, postural muscles. Critically, this is done in functional positions (often standing), and so the transfer of this neuromuscular reprogramming is good.

So far then, it all seems very positive. However, in my view there is still much ground to be made in the application of yoga in football. It was, and still frequently is the case now, that the approach to utilising the benefits of yoga is simply to bring a yoga instructor into the club and ask them to put sessions on. Twenty years ago it was acceptable to bring in a weightlifting coach and simply give them a remit of getting the players stronger. Clearly we have now moved on dramatically from such a clumsy approach, and yet we remain anchored to this way of working with yoga. This is problematic for a number of reasons. Yoga is essentially an element of S&C if we work from our earlier definition of 'physical preparation of athletes'. Consequently it should be applied with the same level of rigour as other methods, and be delivered in a bespoke manner. This means individual prescription is required and should be based on interlinking conversations with other practitioners. These conversations should lead to sessions which target the specific mechanical requirements of the player. Unfortunately many yoga teachers coach towards a fixed technical model rather than 'customising' it to the player. This can be dangerous in high-performance sport as often a player may increase their risk of injury if flexibility is increased too much, particularly if this is not matched with increased strength through range. This is no different from the need to provide subtle adaptations to barbell techniques described previously. Finally, by sticking with the traditional

'yoga class' format we end up with clumsy solutions whereby you either 'do yoga' or you don't. The time available to a player, particularly pre- and post-training, is limited. For a programme to be truly optimal it must be multi-faceted and include many elements. Each of these elements, including yoga, must be able to be distilled down to the essential parts to ensure efficiency and allow the player to move onto the next element.

So why does this not happen? Personally I feel that yoga practitioners and science & medicine teams are divided by a common language. Each will frequently use similar anatomical terms but often with critical differences in meaning, thus causing confusion. Alternatively the language can sometimes have no commonality and therefore communication is difficult. Over the years I have tried to overcome these barriers and build up an understanding with yoga instructors in order to get the most from these powerful tools. One of the more fruitful outcomes of this process was a cross-referenced database of poses against the physical outcome they can be used to target. This is outlined in Table 4.1.

For those interested in incorporating yoga into their practice I would recommend working with a good, open-minded instructor to follow a similar process which allows you both to have a good dialogue. As with any form of exercise (and it goes without saying) that if you wish to coach it, or even understand it, then you need to do it. Experiencing the poses will undoubtedly provide greater insight.

Finally, I personally have found Iyengar yoga to be most effective and appropriate for sports people. Iyengar yoga uses so-called 'props' such as foam bricks, ropes and supports to assist in the pose. This is crucial as far too often players are not flexible enough to produce the desired

Table 4.1   **Yoga Physical Outcomes**

		1/2 Uttan	Downward Dog	Sun Salutes	Half Moon	Hal asana	Parsvottansana	Warrior 3	Tree Pose	Prayer, Cow & Eagle	Trap traction	Headstand	Triangle	Warrior 2	Mountain Pose
Stretches	Posterior Chain	•	•	•	•	•	•	•							
	Traction	•													
	Thoracic Extension		•	•					•	•	•				
	Neural Floss		•			•						•			
	Dorsi-Flexors		•	•											
	Hip Flexors			•			•						•		
	Internal Rotators (hip)				•		•		•				•	•	
	Superficial Front Line												•		
	Lateral Line						•						•		
	Thoracic Rotation						•								
	Rotator Cuff									•	•				
	Pectorals & Deltoid														
	Scapula Control	•	•												
	Scapula Retraction														•
Strengthening	Intrinsic Foot								•						
	Single-leg Stability								•						
	Global Postural Control								•						
	External Rotators (hip)				•				•						
	Posterior Chain							•							

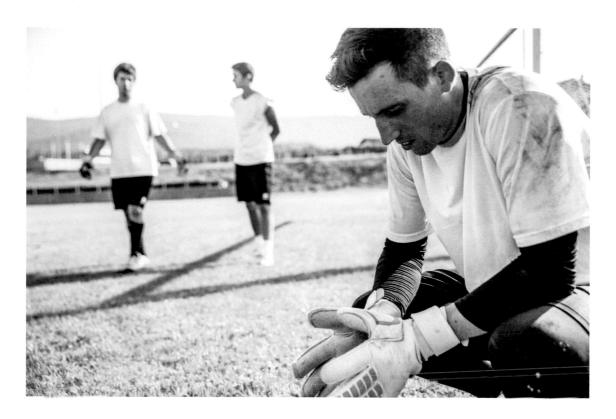

shape and have to compensate by getting movement from another area. This not only makes it ineffective but is also actually likely to take the player backwards, and reinforces poor movement patterns.

4.7 Specific Mobilisation Techniques

To be clear, my tool of choice for improving mobility is the use of moderately loaded, well-chosen and coached barbell movements. However, there are a raft of other tools at our disposal to enable us to have a great deal of efficacy and precision when seeking to improve mobility of a specific joint or structure.

Over the past 10–15 years the use of trigger point release and self-massage tools, such as foam rollers and hockey balls, have significantly enhanced S&C coaches' ability to improve movement beyond simply stretching. It should be noted that while their efficacy is generally accepted, the mechanism behind these tools is still up for debate. Some suggest that 'tissue quality' is enhanced, whereas others believe that the effect is chiefly on the nervous system and pain modulation. As coaches we should always seek to understand the nature of adaptation and not just the effect. Therefore much more insight is required here.

These are supported by neural-flossing techniques which often address the issue of excessive tension which is sometimes mistaken for a lack of length. I have seen many track-and-field athletes arrive complaining of feeling tight but can still move through excellent ranges.

In the past couple of years a practitioner by the name of Kelly Starrett has changed the game dramatically. In his book, *Becoming a Supple Leopard*, Starrett describes the movement and mobility system which gained him notoriety through his website www.mobilityWOD.com. This system uses a comprehensive range of techniques with names as exotic as the title of his book. These include Pressure Wave, Smash & Floss and Voodoo Wrapping. Don't be fooled by the slightly Hollywood nature of these names though. The system he describes is well thought out and backed by reasoned argument and an excellent understanding of movement. Given that my philosophy of effective S&C practice is underpinned by a belief that we get the most from our athletes by making them move better, this system is potentially of huge value to any coach who cares to take the time to embrace and understand it.

4.8 Blood-Flow Restricted Exercise (BFRE)

BFRE, also sometimes described as occlusion or Kaatsu training, has become firmly established as a key tool in S&C rehab in recent years. Essentially this is a technique which aims to increase the metabolic stress on muscle tissue for a given mechanical load by significantly limiting the ability of the body to deliver re-oxygenated blood. This becomes highly valuable in the load-compromised player. Typically a player will either be rehabbing following an injury, and not be able to tolerate the normal mechanical load required to stimulate adaptation optimally, or be long-term compromised through an issue such as osteochondral defects.

In such situations, BFRE has been shown to be highly effective. Over the past few years the mechanisms by which BFRE work have received significant attention in the strength science literature. A summary of the current research is presented in Table 4.2 opposite.

The return to training following serious injury is significantly limited by the time taken to reverse the atrophy suffered during inactivity. By providing us with a means of rebuilding tissue and regaining force production earlier and more quickly, we are empowered to provide a superior rehab. A great example of this can be seen in a study which used passive occlusion (i.e. patients wore the cuff but did not exercise) just three days after an ACL reconstruction up to day 14. The amount of reduction in muscle size was around half that of the controls (20% versus 9%). Of course, the nature of BFRE means that caution should be used and medical approval should always be sought, particularly in an injured athlete. The following basic points should be a bare minimum if you are considering employing these techniques:

- Establish exclusion criteria with medical staff, and check player suitability

- Develop clearly defined protocols with medical staff

- Familiarise the player with the feeling of occlusion before adding exercise (it doesn't feel very nice)

- I would suggest using conservative cuff pressures. Many studies use very high pressures (⋯⟩220mmHg). In my experience and from discussing with colleagues, far lower pressures than this are still effective. There certainly does not appear to be a linear pressure-to-results relationship.

Table 4.2	Overview of BFRE Literature	
		Study
Low-load resistance exercise (~20–50% of 1RM) in combination with blood-flow restriction (BFR) by the use of pressure cuffs has repeatedly been shown to increase muscle strength and cross-sectional area		Moore et al., 2004
During BFRE at 30% of 1RM in the knee-extension exercise, EMG of the quadriceps during the concentric phase reached values close to 100% of MVC during sets near the point of task failure		Wernborn, 2012
With similar lactate responses occluded training may elicit greater growth hormone responses vs. regular training		Reeves et al., 2006, Takarada, 2000
Muscle damage may be lower during occluded training and this may allow for more frequent doses than traditional training		Wernborn, 2012
mTOR has been shown to be elevated 1–3hrs post-training and may last up to 24hrs. This should be considered when planning other training and dose frequency		Wernborn, 2012
Hyperactivation of myogenic satellite cells occurs with blood-flow restricted exercise		Aagaard, 2012
Strength gains of 26% have been shown in elite injured athletes over a 9-day training period with various training protocols		Rosenblatt, 2012
Passive occlusion may attenuate post-operative muscular atrophy by approx 50% over a 2-week period		Takarada, 2000
It appears that benefits of occluded training may also be replicated systemically by exercising in a hypoxic environment		Nishimura, 2010, Kon, 2012

4.9 Summary

We have covered a great deal of ground looking at a model of injury prevention, and yet we are still to name an exercise or deal with the specifics of a single injury. Hopefully this helps to illustrate several key points. Reducing injuries in a squad of players is not easy. To be done effectively it requires contributions from everyone within the system, and these contributions to be coordinated and collaborative to avoid a great deal of wasted effort. Even when we boil it down to the part which we have most control over – exercise interventions – it is not so much about having brilliant exercises but about understanding the exact needs of the individual, what adaptations you need to elicit, and being skilled enough to use a range of tools to achieve them.

005
planning injury prevention

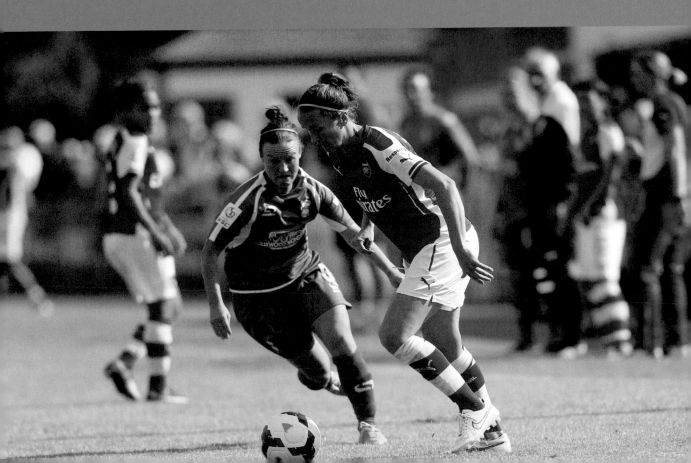

Now that we have considered our philosophy, defined our model of injury prevention and all of the elements within, we now require something to guide us as to which injuries we are going to try to prevent and in whom. As we stated in the conclusion of the previous chapter, one of our key determinants of success will be our ability to know exactly what we are trying to achieve. Consequently, the need to identify where risk and weakness lie is critical.

It is possible to take an epidemiological approach to this question and review the literature regarding injury incidence. This will quickly draw us to obvious conclusions such as the predominance of hamstring, knee and ankle injuries. It may also provide some insight into population-specific concerns such as the increased risk of ACL injury in female players, the heightened risk in competitive games for professionals, and the lower severity of injury in youth players. However, all of these population-specific trends should only ever be considered secondary to the profile of the individual. Therefore our focus is on a broad and thorough assessment of risk.

5.1 Assessment of Risk Part 1 – Conditioning Assessments

Perhaps the most blissfully uncomplicated element of risk assessment comes from the measure of muscular capacity. When assessing movement qualities, there are a galaxy of possible dysfunctions and interactions which must then be applied to an infinite number of movement challenges. If I am tight here, will it affect my apparent instability there? If I see this movement in isolation, can I be sure it will remain the same in a complex pattern? Consequently, estimating (let alone calculating) the burden a given structure will face is a mammoth task. When measuring capacity

though we simply need to produce tests which will identify how much we can produce (or tolerate), compare it to relevant normative data, and use it as a benchmark to assess the efficacy of our attempts to improve it through training.

Capacity testing has enjoyed something of a renaissance in recent years. The rise in popularity of functional movement screens meant that capacity testing had become rather unfashionable. However, it became clear that while we were able to gain insight into movement control of players, we knew little of their ability to tolerate load or resist fatigue. Consequently we have emerged with a common-sense view whereby movement quality and capacity assessment sit side-by-side and complement each other. There are limitations to these tests of course. They are very much a blunt instrument and are only intended to give a broad overview. Critics point out that specific elements of musculature cannot be assessed and so weakness cannot be pinpointed. The nature of the tests is not always particularly 'functional' either. Both true. However, rather than dispense with them this simply means that we acknowledge that they merely represent another part of the puzzle rather than providing the whole answer when assessing risk.

Ideally these tests do not sit within the programme as isolated testing tools, but instead are exercises which are used regularly in training and therefore the player is familiarised with. This not only adds to the reliability of the test but also reduces the risk of an adverse delayed onset muscle soreness (DOMS) reaction to maximal testing. The tests below are examples which are relevant to common injuries and that I have found insightful in my practice. However, they are neither mandatory nor exclusive. The main criteria for an exercise test being suitable are that you can be confident that it targets the intended musculature and that the point of failure is within an appropriate time frame and results from capacity (rather than pain, boredom, loss of skill, etc.). It should be acknowledged that the validity and reliability of these tests also relies very much on player motivation and willingness to work hard. For this reason it can be useful to impose minimal standards. Failure to achieve these results in additional training to reach the standard. This is especially effective when players are not previously informed of the level they need to achieve.

An interesting question to ask when conducting these types of test is exactly what are we measuring – fitness or fatigue? This became apparent to during a bout of pre-season testing. Having used many of these tests as exercises during the previous season, I had a good idea of the numbers most players were capable of producing. Tests were scheduled to see how much the players had lost during the summer. Consequently it was a surprise to see that, to a man, they all produced more on the first day back in training than they had at any point in the previous season. As much as I would have loved to think that this was down to their summer diligence and adherence to my methods, this would be utterly delusional. Instead it provided me with a priceless insight into the nature of exactly what was limiting players in-season. Clearly conditioning gains in the gym were being masked by residual fatigue. Once again this highlights the fact that injury risk is a beast of many limbs.

Hamstring Bridge Test
If there is one muscle group which medical departments universally seek to protect it is surely the hamstrings. The single-leg hamstring bridge is

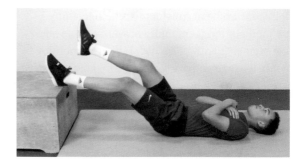

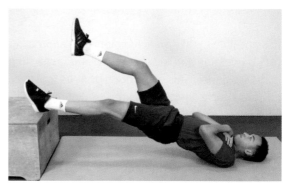

Hamstring Bridge Test

a simple exercise which tests the capacity of the hamstrings to produce hip extension in a reasonably functional position. This has been shown to be predictive of hamstring injuries in Australian Rule Football players.

The test uses a 60cm box, with the heel of the leg to be tested placed on the top with a slight bend in the knee. The hips are lifted off the floor by pushing through the heel. The free leg should be kept bent and must not be swung to assist the movement. The tester places a hand at the top of the movement to ensure that the hip has been extended for each rep with the touch on the floor representing the bottom of the movement. Reps are performed every 2 seconds until the player cannot continue. It is worth noting that both a low absolute score, or a low score relative to the opposite leg are risk factors for injury.

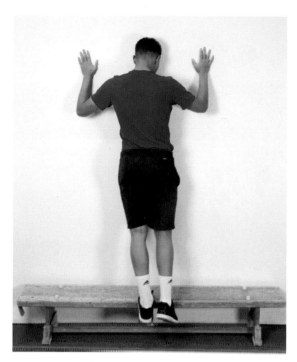

Calf-Raise Test

Of course, many medical departments use an isokinetic assessment of hamstrings (through knee flexion rather than hip extension). This has pros and cons. The data is much more detailed as the production of force through the range is described. The validity of this can depend upon the speed of movement though. The test certainly provides some level of normative benchmark for players who sustain a hamstring injury. I have also seen skilled physios identify other issues around the knee during screening when picking up anomalies in the force trace. The critics of the test point out that the position, and nature of the movement, are non-functional. Interestingly, Bennel and colleagues did not find this test to be predictive of injury in a study of over 100 Australian Rule Footballers. Therefore I would suggest that these tests should not be viewed as replication as they offer very distinct advantages over one another.

Calf-Raise Test

The triceps surae muscle-tendon unit, or the calf and Achilles tendon in lay terms, are another area which frequently break down under the stress of training and playing. The repeated calf-raise test is an effective way of assessing this area.

The test is performed by placing the ball of the foot on a step or small box. Hands are placed lightly on a support for balance only (best to insist on fingertip contact). The player begins at the bottom of the range in full plantar flexion and then raises and lowers to a 2s tempo, with full control and even pace throughout. This test can induce significant DOMS if unfamiliar, so I suggest using it with caution in training and to avoid introducing it at the start of pre-season testing.

Trunk-Capacity Tests

The ability of the trunk to resist unwanted movement has implications for a vast array of injuries, both locally and globally. I have deliberately avoided using the word 'core' as it is plagued by misunderstanding and misrepresentation.

The **isometric back-extension test**, or Sorensen test, measures the ability to resist spinal flexion

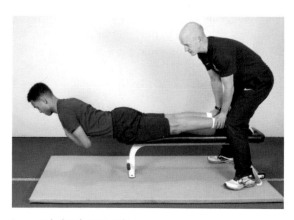

Isometric back-extension test

and has been shown to be a predictor of lower back pain.

The lower body is fixed by a partner or tester to a bench or plinth. The bench should fall just below the iliac crest. The arms should be placed across the chest. The trunk, neck and head are held parallel to the ground and the time that this position can be maintained is recorded. The test is ended when the torso drops below parallel, or immediately in the presence of pain. The position is held as long as possible up to a maximum of 240 seconds.

The **side plank** is a very common gym exercise. It is effective as a gym exercise as it maximally recruits the musculature involved in preventing lateral flexion. For the same reason, it serves as an effective test of the same qualities.

The body is held in a fixed position with each segment kept in line. The feet can either be held on top of each other or with one behind the other. The elbow is placed beneath the shoulder. The player holds the position as long as they can maintain. Ensure that the shoulder does not hitch toward the ear and that the hips do not sag.

The **double-leg lower** test provides a relatively functional challenge to the anterior trunk in that it must resist extension while allow movement of the lower limbs.

Lying prone, the player brings the medial malleolus of one ankle level with the lateral epicondyle of the opposite knee. The thigh angle of the bent leg represents the top of the movement. That leg is then extended and the opposite leg finally lifted to the same angle. To perform a repetition, the legs are then lowered in a controlled fashion to give a light touch on the floor before returning to the

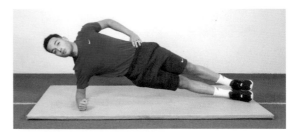

Side plank

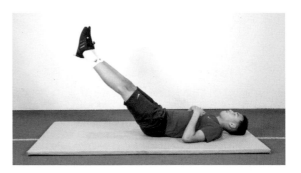

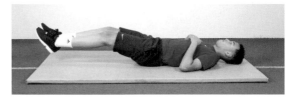

Double-leg Lower Test

start. The test finishes when the player cannot perform any more repetitions, or if they are unable to maintain a neutral lumbar spine (i.e. when they are moving into greater extension). This may be monitored either through palpation or the use of a pressure cuff.

Normative Scores

The scores below in Table 5.1 are typical of what I have seen in elite football populations. I would suggest that these tests be viewed as players needing to achieve a threshold, beyond which there are diminishing returns. I believe it is a mistake to treat these as if there is a dose response. If you have injury concerns with a player and they achieve the normative threshold, or mildly exceed it, then the likelihood is that vulnerability lies elsewhere and this is where your efforts are best directed.

5.2 Assessment of Risk Part 2 – Movement Assessment

Given that I have stated that my philosophy is based primarily on improving quality of movement, it is imperative that I have a method of assessing both the starting point and the effects of my interventions.

It is very rare to find an SSM department which does not conduct a formalised functional movement screening (FMS) of some sort. These started life fairly homogeneously through the work of Gray Cook, and have evolved in that some still stick with branded movement screen, whereas others have adapted the tests and the way in which they are assessed to produce a more bespoke protocol. For some reason the subject of movement screening is one which tends to divide

our profession like no other. Some swear by it, others swear about it. I think it is important not to be overly dogmatic and tribal about these things though. My personal preference is to be able to work with players closely enough that I get to see their movement qualities in the gym all the time. I therefore do not need additional tests, as I am able to regularly monitor and evaluate acute and chronic changes in movement capacity. However, I equally recognise that when working with large squads and a small staff this is a very convenient way of quantifying a broad picture of how well a player moves. You will have to decide for yourself which method fits your own particular working situation.

We could fill all the remaining pages of this book and beyond with discussion around each of the various tests, the dysfunctions which we are looking for and potential solutions. Instead, I think it is more useful to give consideration to exactly what we are trying to evaluate. If you wish to learn more about the assessment of dysfunction I would direct you towards the excellent book by Shirley Sahrmann – *Diagnosis and Treatment of Movement Impairment Syndromes*.

Table 5.1	Normative Conditioning Assessment Scores	
Test	**Mean Score**	**Comment**
Hamstring Bridge	40±11*	L vs. R ratio of 0.95
Calf Raise	30±5	
Isometric Back-Extension	150s±22	Maximum of 240s
Side Plank	120s±23	
Double-Leg Lower	41±17	Control limiting factor approx. 50% of cases

* This is taken from pre-season data. In-season I have typically used a target of 30 repetitions.

I would generally begin any assessment with a review of standing posture. This tells us how everything 'hangs together'. This also provides important clues as to limiting factors. If structures are restricted and begin in poor positions, the chances of an ideal movement being produced are practically nil. This also steers us away from neural control and closer to structural interventions.

I like to use a bilateral-squat challenge to assess global mobility. Principally this provides information around mobility of ankles, hips and thoracic spine. In extreme cases this can also test stability of knees and trunk. When the global movement pattern is compromised this then leads us to further, more local assessment. The test may come in the form of back squat, front squat or bodyweight squat. Which one you use comes down to a personal preference and the abilities and dimensions of the player. The addition of an overhead squat provides very useful insight into thoracic mobility, which, as we have discussed previously, can have important implications for the whole of the posterior chain.

If bilateral movement predominantly informs about mobility, the challenge to stability comes from unilateral exercises. This begins with a controlled movement exercise such as a lunge or single-leg squat. Of course, while unwanted movement is typically seen at the knee, it is much more common that the source of the instability comes from the hip or the ankle. These controlled movements require a combination of strength and skill to control positions. We also need to move to more skill-based challenges which test the ability to exhibit neuromuscular control during dynamic situations. This will come in the form of some level of hopping and landing task, such as the hop-stick exercise. The key is that it must involve a landing element and be dynamic enough to test the player's ability to resist falling into knee valgus. I would suggest that both in training and testing this task should be varied to ensure that it is testing control as a true ability rather than the specific skill of one particular exercise. Many coaches also like to use a star-excursion test, which provides a more varied assessment of dynamic knee stability.

It could be argued that the functional nature of the double-leg lower test from the conditioning assessment battery provides a measure of trunk stability. I would look at this as a relatively high-level challenge and therefore like to include a lower-level challenge. Over the years I have found the dead bug exercise to be very insightful. This relatively easy task demands lumbo-pelvic control during diagonal, alternate limb movement patterns. While almost any player can perform the task, where they feel the work is generated can vary greatly. Those who feel no effort or that the work comes from the external obliques (aka lower abdominals) are not a concern. However, some will report that they feel the work coming from their back. This is a significant red flag in my experience as it represents a failure to recruit the appropriate, deep stabilising musculature in a low-level task. Anecdotally, I have found strong correlations between this 'dysfunction' and groin injury.

An aspect of movement assessment which is not so commonly applied is the observation of movement during play. This can be a very enlightening process. If isolated musculoskeletal screening highlights potential movement issues, and movement screening tests whether these are present in functional tasks, then observation of play gives us the truest test of whether there is actually an issue. Of course, this process is not without its difficulties. The high-speed, multi-

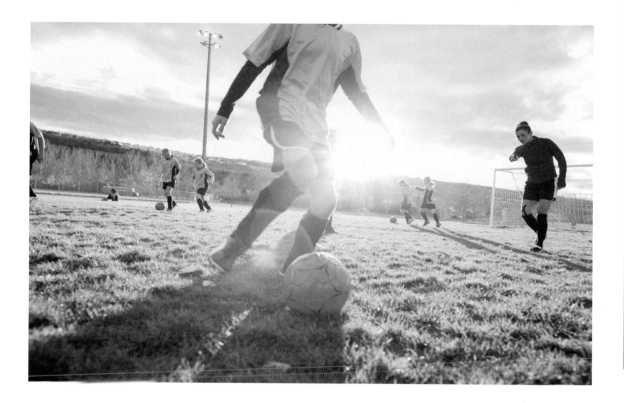

directional and chaotic nature of play means that specific movements are difficult to isolate. If this was the only movement assessment tool used then it would also be impossible to determine the root cause of any movement issue seen. However, when this 'big picture' is combined with the isolated knowledge acquired through more controlled interventions (i.e. MSK and FMS), then the team is able to get a very rounded and insightful view of injury risk and the issues behind it.

In practical terms I would recommend that this approach is best used on targeted players in targeted movements. For example, a winger who often injures a hamstring during high-speed running may have their mechanics assessed in play (which is typically very different to just asking them to sprint in isolation). Alternatively, a player who appears to suffer valgus collapse of

the knee in an FMS task may be reviewed during change of direction challenges to gauge risk of ACL and other injuries.

5.3 Assessment of Risk Part 3 – Abstract Factors

Our model of injury prevention is based on the premise that risk is reduced by a combination of reducing the mechanical burden on tissues (improving movement efficiency) and increasing tissue tolerance. This philosophy underpins the content of most medical and sports science screening processes. However, it is also worth considering that there may be some more abstract aspects of a player's make-up which play a role in contributing to their injury risk. The model shown in Figure 5.1 below considers a number of factors which are often overlooked, yet can be key in pushing a player into a high-risk situation. It is worth noting that this model was formed off the back of a lively debate over coffee one afternoon with Matt Green and Chris Barnes (two excellent sports scientists). It is these conversations with forward-thinking people that often act as far more important CPD than conferences and books.

Acute Changes

Insufficient conditioning is a fairly obvious reason why a player's risk would increase. Most clubs are now fairly alert to the need to add training volume to players who, usually through non-selection, have dropped below the required fitness levels. What is less obvious is the risk of a **different training regime**. I have seen on numerous occasions a new head coach will join the club and overhaul the training schedule. In terms of absolute numbers this may not look very different. However, while the amount of training may be similar, the change in physical demands, brought about very suddenly, can put the player at high risk. This is exacerbated when the nature of their role in the team also changes.

Technical overload occurs when a player is required to perform technically or tactically to a level which stretches them excessively. There are a number of factors which contribute to this. Anxiety may occur when the player becomes technically uncomfortable, leading to an increase in muscular tension. It is also likely that the player will find themselves in situations where they are reacting later than usual or reaching to make up for an error. Young players moving up into the senior squad are particularly at risk of this problem. This is a great example of an abstract risk factor which may not be measured in normal training metrics. In such cases the value of having someone watch training with a purpose and talking to the rest of the team is vital.

Training Behaviour

Being either a **high-load** or a **low-load** player can been seen as a risk factor. By the term 'loading' I am referring to the mechanical burden a player typically accumulates in their training and playing profile (through accelerometer data). This is not a factor of their weight, but is a combination of the

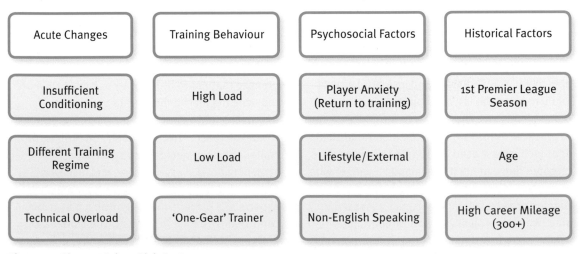

Acute Changes	Training Behaviour	Psychosocial Factors	Historical Factors
Insufficient Conditioning	High Load	Player Anxiety (Return to training)	1st Premier League Season
Different Training Regime	Low Load	Lifestyle/External	Age
Technical Overload	'One-Gear' Trainer	Non-English Speaking	High Career Mileage (300+)

Figure 5.1 Abstract Injury Risk Factors

nature of their locomotion and the efficiency with which movements are executed. For example, some players will accumulate lots of load through many rapid changes of direction, whereas others tend to run in straight lines and curves. Similarly, some are very efficient and change direction without huge mechanical load, whereas others are much less effective. Great movers such as Lionel Messi and Zlatan Ibrahimovic are good examples of the former. It may seem surprising to consider a low-load player to be at risk. However, we have found that because these players only have a low exposure to load, a modest increase in absolute load represents a big increase in relative load. Clearly this represents a dangerous situation when a player faces unfamiliar physical burden.

The concept of a **one-gear trainer** is one which raises some interesting moral questions around training application. If a player is too 'honest' in training they may not be being particularly smart. Players who pride themselves in always giving their best can often inadvertently end up with a training regime which is not effectively periodised – they go all-out every time. On the flip side, there are players who, in football parlance, know how to 'look after themselves'. Essentially this means that if they feel like they need an easier day they are willing and able to drop down the gears and hide a little in training. This might not necessarily sit well with the ethos of commitment and passion, but in reality, these players often do the medical department a big favour.

Psychosocial Factors

One factor which came to light during a particularly tricky rehab and subsequent re-injury is **player anxiety**, particularly during return to training. As a department, we found that despite being able to achieve all of our return-to-play markers in rehab and perform to a good level, this player would continually re-injure when he joined squad training. What was curious was that the injuries were occurring early on and during apparently innocuous tasks. After lots of soul searching, inquiry and conversations with the player it became clear that the way he psychologically processed being back with the squad was very different to isolated rehab. Subsequently his self-induced anxiety was causing him to become dangerously tight and vulnerable. As a result of this experience we changed our return-to-play protocols for medium to long-term injuries. These now had opportunities to take part in the squad warm-up before breaking away to conduct end stage rehab (thus gently re-introducing). We also started to make more use of the young pro groups as a stepping stone to full training.

In a similar vein but much more broadly, the player's **lifestyle and external** issues can be a very significant risk factor for injury. Some examples are obvious, such as the dangers of enjoying the nightlife too much. However, life challenges such as having a baby in the house (with disturbed sleep, stressed partner, etc.), sick relatives, and all of the other things which bring stress into the lives of the rest of us, also affect footballers. In order to be able to take these elements into consideration and react accordingly it is vital to have good relationships with players. This does not mean being their best friend, but there must be informal lines of communication (which can take many forms) to ensure that this important information is picked up.

The presence of **non-English speaking** players is no longer simply a Premier League phenomenon. Players not just from Europe but around the world now participate across the leagues in England. Of course, many arrive with good English already. However, if they do not have at least a working knowledge of the language it can be a real problem. This comes from the difficulty in communicating small sensitivities. If a player is 'yellow flagged', the pre-training informal questioning can form a key element in the decision as to whether or not they are restricted, or even removed from training. Without good communication this process can easily fall down. In such circumstances, Google Translate can be a very valuable tool. It is also hugely helpful to have another player who can translate and they are close to. Interestingly, it has been shown that the successful transfer of a player from one environment to another is much more likely if some of their colleagues are brought with them (be it medical staff, a player, etc.). If you are lucky enough to be able to influence such decisions, this may be worth considering when investing in foreign players.

Historical Factors

At the risk of making this section Anglocentric, we have observed a significant injury risk during a player's **first season in the Premier League** (much reduced in subsequent seasons). On reflection, and based on the physical data we have already seen in previous chapters, it may be that this is not a product of the Premier League being unprecedentedly hard, but instead just that it is unique and thus represents an unaccustomed physical and technical challenge. Consequently it may well be the case that a move between any two leagues where there is an up-regulation in either physical or technical demands will create a similar risk.

We cannot ignore a **player's age** as, despite conditioning methods and anomalies such as Giggs and Maldini, sadly our ability to recover and regenerate declines with age. As these two examples demonstrate though, it is certainly possible to mediate against this with sensible

lifestyle management and adaptation of playing role (plus good S&C of course). This is distinct from **career mileage** though. Anyone who has worked in the game will know that football is attritional. There are young men in the game who have played volumes of football beyond their years – and it shows. Similarly, players who come into the game later can often go beyond our expectations and are still relatively well functioning in their 30s. Of course not all football is created equally. Very high volumes at a young age are likely to be more damaging than a more sensible progressive increase. This is often a reflection of the ability of sports scientists and Academy coaches to work together to produce an intelligent development plan for the most talented players who are at risk of being overused.

In practical terms, assimilating all of these abstract factors to a point whereby they allow you to make practical decisions can seem intimidating (as can be the case with traditional assessments as we will soon discuss). A very simple but effective method of doing so is to score each element out of 3 to produce a risk index. You may wish to make this more sensitive and add a weighting scale to place greater emphasis on one category over another. However, there is a risk that this may overcomplicate things, and there is evidence to suggest that non-weighted systems are just as powerful. An example of a suitable table is given above.

5.4 Assessment of Risk Part 4 – Bringing in the Medics and Pulling it all Together

So far we have discussed conditioning assessments, movement assessments and abstract injury risks. This already represents a mass of data before we even begin to consider the metabolic conditioning assessments carried out by

Table 5.2	Abstract Risk Index Calculator			
Risk Factor	**Category Weighting**	**Risk Level**		
		High (3)	**Moderate (2)**	**Low (1)**
Insufficient conditioning				
Different training regime				
Technical overload				
High load				
Low load				
One gear trainer				
Player anxiety (RTT)				
Lifestyle/external				
Non-English speaking				
New to league				
Age				
High career mileage				

sports science staff and the comprehensive musculoskeletal (MSK) tests performed by the medics. When combined, this results in an ocean of data to assess and, critically, respond to. To make matters worse the bulk of this work tends to be carried out during the beginning of the pre-season period when training volume is high and time is most limited. While the world has fallen in love with so-called 'big data', it is only powerful when you can do something meaningful with it.

Perfectionism can be a dangerous trap in such situations. The desire to constantly add insightful tests or tweak existing ones to make them slightly better can completely undermine the whole process. In my personal view, I believe the most effective approach is to encourage all involved to be as lean and consistent in their test selection as possible. A small number of tests which you understand intimately and can track and compare historically are far more powerful than an ever changing raft of procedures on which you cannot act with the confidence of historical proof.

A possible challenge to achieving such a philosophy comes from the desire of so many to replicate their own version of the fabled 'Milan Lab'. This was the project run by AC Milan from 2002 and headed-up by Jean-Pierre Meersseman, with the intention of predicting and reducing injury risk. Credited with having extended the careers of stars such as Paolo Maldini and Alessandro Costacurta into their 40s, this is clearly something any football club would wish to emulate. The method of the Milan Lab is based upon the collection of masses of data from all kinds of areas, and the statistical processing to calculate risk and inform interventions. However, it is the statistical analysis which is generally either overlooked entirely, or not performed with sufficient power or insight, which tends to cause attempts at replication to fall flat. Consequently there is a growing trend for statistical analysis to be outsourced to genuine experts. I was fortunate enough to work briefly with the late and brilliant Nick Broad when he was at PSG. Here I saw a first-class example of such a process with all manner of data sent to a statistics expert which was then woven into the fabric of how training was constructed. This was a very rare example of truly world-class practice from a man who is still sorely missed within the game.

I would certainly not profess to be anything remotely close to a statistics expert. However, recent experience has led me to the conclusion that, for those brave enough to embrace it, Bayesian statistics may be the missing link which holds the key to replicating the success of the Milanese. This methodology has re-emerged in recent years to become somewhat *en vogue* (if statistics can ever be described as fashionable). I will not attempt to give any kind of meaningful explanation of this complex theory but in essence it differs from traditional approaches in that it makes heavy use of prior knowledge of a situation and subjective expert view to make predictions. If you do decide to explore this further I would urge you to utilise external expertise. Be warned though, to properly build this model is a long and complex process, it won't solve your problems tomorrow or even this season.

In the absence of world-class statistical insight and the avoidance of superfluous data, how best can we maximise the impact of our streamlined injury risk assessment data? As simplistic as it may sound, instinct may be the key. If I were to ask you to name the top five players most at risk of injury in the forthcoming season, my guess is that you would end up at least 80% right when days lost to injury are calculated at the end of the season. The only exception to this is likely to be when a player suffers an unpredictable serious contact injury. What is more, I suspect that you would also be able to have a pretty good stab at identifying the nature of the injuries which will keep these players out of games and training. I firmly believe that it is how you support this critical mass which will chiefly determine your impact on days lost over the course of the year. Of course, this does not mean that nobody else receives attention. Rather, the top concerns need to be case studied and provided with highly bespoke management programmes. Five 2-hour case conferences, where all the aspects of risk assessment can be discussed, can be highly productive. This is simply not possible for a 24-player squad, nor is the delivery of the individualised management. Therefore the mass of data collected is still available for reference for all players when required and to provide baselines for injury. However, it becomes streamlined in terms of managing it as the in-depth analysis and debate is only required for a much smaller number.

5.5 Periodisation of Injury Prevention

Is there merit in shifting the focus of injury prevention systems throughout specific stages of the season? On the face of it there may be some logic to this. Those in the game will often express the view that pre-season and the early competitive season represent high-risk periods for tendon

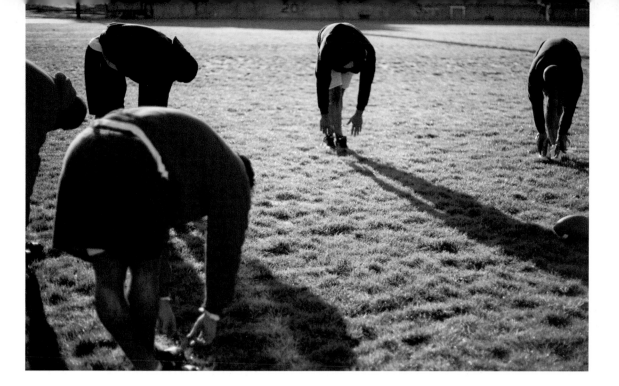

injury. This certainly has a logical basis, given what we have learned regarding tendons and the need for regular mechanical loading in Chapter 4. The potential negative consequence of de-loading tendons during the off-season, combined with firmer pitches during July and August, plus high running volumes in pre-season all support this view. The received wisdom holds that the risk to tendons dissipates as training is accumulated. The burden then shifts to muscular injuries as we move towards Christmas and January. Again, the logic here is sound as residual fatigue begins to accumulate, temperatures drop and games come thick and fast (certainly in the English leagues). This trend of early tendon risk moving towards muscular priority has been supported by a study of a Spanish team over two seasons.

In full confidence of this logical hypothesis I have attempted to apply a specific analysis of the injury data over several seasons with squads I have worked with. However, to my surprise, no genuine trends were evident. Even when injuries have clustered it is hard to establish a genuine trend rather than coincidence. (This is a real problem as three similar injuries are often treated as a trend which must be solved, when the law of averages suggests that this is likely to be simply a mathematical cluster.) So perhaps I can suggest a slight amendment to the conventional wisdom. Maybe it is more insightful to say that during the early season, the players who tend to have tendon issues will suffer their injuries predominantly at this time. Likewise, those who typically suffer muscular injuries will pick up their problems during the winter. Consequently, over the years I have come to take the following view with regard to periodisation, that your own individual weaknesses will crack when your own individual threshold is exceeded.

The nature of the training will also have a significant impact, specifically whether the work is intensive (small spaces) or extensive (larger spaces). However, there is no automatic link between each of these and a phase of the season.

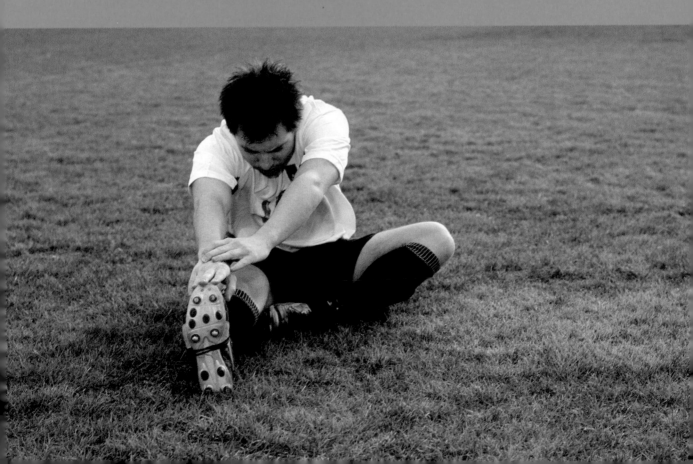

006
specific injury-prevention systems: hamstrings

Over the years I have come to learn that one of the key characteristics of a successful S&C coach is the possession of a system. This system may be simple or complex, driven by literature or experience, written or simply known. Regardless, it must have logic, be understood by the coach and, critically, repeatable and adaptable.

The following specific injury prevention systems are my own blend of art and science which I have found to be effective over the years. Once again, these are essentially a philosophy. They may serve as a starting point for a thought process, be applied verbatim, or simply used to contrast with your own thoughts to provide greater certainty as to your position on the various debates which surround a topic.

6.1 Hamstring Injury

If birth, death and taxes are the only certainties in life, it could be argued that hamstring injuries hold the same status in football. This is an inherently high-risk injury as is seen across a vast range of running-based sports. The problem seems to be exacerbated by the fact that far too often coaches have sought to solve this highly complex injury dilemma with overly simplistic solutions. A brief web search of the literature will reveal an apparent obsession with proving the efficacy of the Nordic hamstring curl (or other similar eccentric training methods) on reducing injury incidence. These generally show that such methods can be effective – although maybe we shouldn't be too shocked to learn that stronger muscles are more robust than weak muscles. As we will see, this is very far from being the whole picture when it comes to reducing risk.

Hamstring injury risk is hugely multi-factorial. As a consequence, managing risk in a given player involves dealing with a unique blend of many factors. It is therefore only appropriate that the system outlined in Table 6.1 is best described as an overview of all the factors to consider as opposed to a recipe to follow. The hamstring system is based on the central principle that injury occurs when stress tolerance is exceeded. Therefore all interventions are directed towards the following goals:

- Reduction of excessive stress through monitoring of training volume and an understanding of individual player thresholds/ fatigue status

- Reduction of hamstring stress through mechanical optimisation

- Enhanced capacity through increased work capacity/fitness

- Enhanced capacity through increased tissue tolerance

The most practical and powerful interventions are those which increase tissue tolerance and control training volume, as these can have quick and definite benefits. Mechanical and movement interventions are important, but the benefits can take time to come to fruition.

6.2 Biomechanical Optimisation

Any programme aimed at optimising the function of the hamstrings ignores the role of the pelvis at its peril. The image in Figure 6.1 (page 63) demonstrates the dramatic role the pelvis plays in hamstring length (and therefore tension and force-production capability).

Table 6.1	Hamstring Injury-Prevention System			
Biomechanical Optimisation	**Movement Patterns**	**Muscle Capacity**	**Muscle Function**	**Stress Modulation**
Optimise pelvic alignment and control	Hip activation and mobility drills in warm-up	Benchmark score of 30 SL Ham Bridge with ⟵···15% LR diff.	Site/Mechanism of injury specific work	Training load monitoring and altering
Optimise glute function (timing and capacity) – beyond remedial	Bespoke preparation for 'at risk' players	End of range eccentric strength in SL (true eccentric)	Reactivity work (various), including kicks	Abstract factors
Inclusion of neural flossing and regular self-slump test	Lumbo-pelvic focussed drills and hamstring coordination	Eccentric strength under fatigue	Opposed & unopposed sprinting for hamstring timing	
Optimal posture and movement through entire posterior chain, including thoracic and cervical spine	Running mechanics interventions to promote correct hamstring use	'Functional lengthening', e.g. Sumos, RDL, Nordics, etc.	Isokinetic profiles of high-risk players established	
	Hip-dominant squat patterns			

This can be addressed from two perspectives. Firstly, there is the static posture. A natural lordosis is very common in sprinters and players blessed with great speed. Paradoxically this may offer a performance advantage as well as increasing injury risk. Consequently much debate exists as to whether one should seek to change this position. What is certainly true is that we should seek to avoid a habit of stabilising the lumbar spine through 'locking' into an anterior-tilted pelvis. Failing to co-contract through both the anterior and posterior musculature has implications for this and a number of other injuries. While the view of ideal may vary between coaches, there should be an awareness of **optimising the pelvic alignment** for a given player. Further consideration should also be given to **pelvic control**. A player may present with perfectly normal pelvic alignment during a standing postural assessment, but a lack of neuromuscular control during running, kicking, etc., may result in the pelvis rapidly moving into uncontrolled anterior tilt (along with other planes of movement). In my view, this player is at greater risk than the player who starts in a position of lordosis but can control it. This view is supported by studies which have shown reductions in hamstring injury incidence

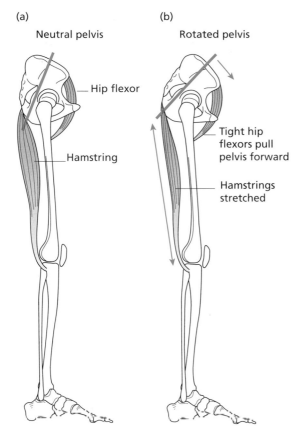

(a) Neutral pelvis

(b) Rotated pelvis

Hip flexor

Hamstring

Tight hip flexors pull pelvis forward

Hamstrings stretched

Figure 6.1 The Role of Pelvic Tilt on Hamstring Length

following the implementation of lumbo-pelvic control training.

We have previously discussed the need to ensure that the hamstrings do not become over-burdened during hip extension if the **glute function** is not optimal. Here it is important that the amount of force produced by the glutes is maximised, but also that the timing of glute firing in the kinetic chain is appropriate. The task of training this low-level motor education will often fall between the S&C coach and the physiotherapist. Once the basic firing sequence has been established (i.e.

glutes recruited prior to hamstrings in a proximo-distal fashion), then it is necessary to take this small spark and develop it into a flame. This is often neglected, or is not fully developed. Those responsible need to take this very basic motor skill and make it as robust as possible. This means developing capacity to ensure that the pattern remains intact when faced with volume and associated fatigue. The pattern must be reproducible during production of high-force movements. It must be consistent during high-speed movements and during a variety of skill tasks. In short, we need to make sure that we haven't simply assumed that a firing sequence seen lying prone in a slow, controlled, low-force movement, will transfer to the field of play. Forgive me if this sounds obvious, but this transition from plinth to pitch is a big area of risk.

For a number of players, the value of addressing neural tissue through techniques such as **neural flossing** can be tremendous. This is particularly common in sprinter-type players. I have lost count of the number of times I have worked with track-and-field athletes who arrive complaining of feeling tight. These same athletes then go on to bring their thigh to their nose as they loosen off. Clearly the hamstrings themselves are not tight. The sensation is arriving from the nerves. Players who tend to report such feelings should become habituated with the performance of a morning slump test. This is a simple process which involves sitting on a bed or bench with a rounded back and the chin on the chest. The legs are then straightened alternately with the ankle dorsi-flexed to check for neural tension through the posterior chain. Sensations of tightness then alert the player to the need to 'floss'. This is a slow, dynamic process which gently mobilises neural tissue. Ensuring that movements are free from such tightness is vital prior to training or playing if risk is to be controlled.

So far we have taken an expansive and holistic view to addressing local biomechanical issues relating to the hamstrings by looking at the role of the pelvis and the glutes. Is that enough though? I would suggest not, as we need to consider the whole of the posterior chain. This includes **thoracic and cervical posture**. The influence of myofascial slings dictates that no element of the chain can be ignored. I have seen real-life examples of players who appear to be healthy in all other aspects of biomechanical optimisation, but still seemed predisposed to hamstring injury. However, these players frequently exhibit poor thoracic posture (i.e. kyphotic, rounded shoulders). This will naturally produce more tension further down the chain, which can sometimes be the difference between health and injury.

6.3 Movement Patterns

If biomechanical optimisation describes our approach to local, isolated posture and motor control, movement patterns reflect the need to incorporate these adaptations into gross movements. We have already looked at the issues which come from an excessive reliance on the hamstrings to produce hip extension where the gluteals are not functioning optimally. Therefore **hip activation and mobility drills** during the warm-up may help to reduce the load through the hamstrings in the subsequent training session or match. Of course, we have touched upon the debate around 'firing the glutes' in Chapter 4. However, it still remains a prudent course of action to utilise multi-directional, whole-body drills to restore range-of-movement and encourage activation of the entire hip complex.

Allied to the above, the promotion of **hip dominant squat patterns** can be very impactful. This is important as a counter to the natural dominance of

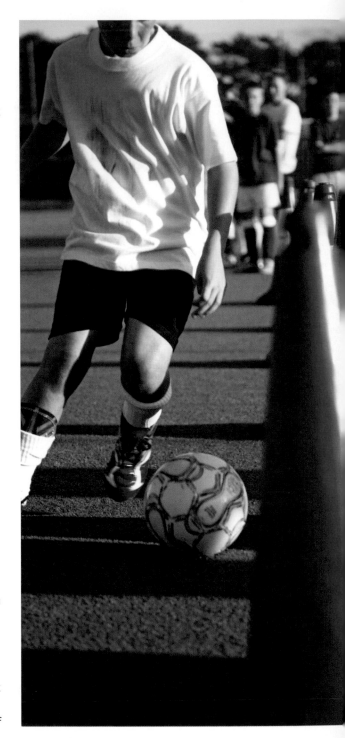

the quadriceps over the hamstring exhibited by most players. As mentioned earlier, the development of low-level glute contribution to hip extension into larger patterns can be a tricky one. The use of good squatting technique to promote this can make the task much simpler. This is a great example of the use of a barbell exercise to promote better movement, as we saw in Chapter 4. Personally, I have found box squats to be very effective in achieving this specific mechanical shift to ensure that there is an increased contribution of the hips to the movement in favour of the knees. Of course, the same can be achieved through appropriate cueing of the exercise, but box squats help to provide consistency, especially when the coach:player ratio is low.

The drills above can realistically be delivered in a generic manner. However, in line with our theory regarding the critical mass of injury risk, at-risk players may benefit from additional **bespoke preparation**. This should be designed to very specifically address any movement dysfunctions or technique issues which may contribute to risk (and are modifiable). For practical reasons, this is probably best delivered prior to commencing the general group warm-up (or as a replacement in extreme cases and where staffing allows).

We have also looked at the importance of low-level control of the pelvis in a localised and isolated manner. However, there is also a need for functional drills which demand **lumbo-pelvic control** during gross, high-speed movements. These can typically be represented by sprint drills from track and field, with a coaching focus placed on maintaining control of the trunk and pelvis. Once again, the environment in which this is coached is as important as the exercise selection. If these are performed without excellent technique they are actually worse than useless,

as the player will inadvertently be rehearsing a poorly controlled movement.

Running mechanics drills will require lumbo-pelvic control, but there will also be a focus on the movements of the lower limb to minimise inappropriate hamstring challenge. Of course, the same exercises may serve to achieve both this and the previous goal, but it should be acknowledged that they are separate outcomes. The most important element of running mechanics is to reduce what has been described as the 'pendulum swing'. At the point of toe-off during the gait cycle, we should aim for simultaneous hip and knee flexion. Typically players will have delayed hip flexion, causing the thigh to come through very late. As a consequence hip extension during the subsequent stride is dominated by concentric use of the hamstrings as opposed to glute maximus. This is a simplification of the mechanical issues involved, but illustrates why a failure to run efficiently causes many players to build up excessive residual fatigue in this muscle group. This is discussed in much more detail in Chapter 10. As an aside, I have found that there are broadly two types of hamstring mechanical risk. There are players blessed with great speed who place huge acute demands on the posterior thigh due to the forces they are required to buffer during sprinting. On the other hand there are the 'plodders' who run in the manner described above, whose hamstrings suffer a long, slow, death.

6.4 Muscle Capacity

So far we have looked at how we can affect movement to reduce the burden on the hamstrings. As we stated at the beginning though, the quickest route to protection comes simply by increasing the capacity of the musculature involved.

During Chapter 5 we discussed **muscle capacity tests**, and specifically the hamstring bridge test. This provides us with two key pieces of information. Firstly, we gain an insight into the endurance of the hamstrings to repeatedly produce force. Secondly, we learn how well balanced this quality is across the left and right limbs. In my experience a target score of 30 repetitions on each leg with a left-right difference no greater than 15% represents a useful and attainable benchmark.

If this appears to be a somewhat general, non-specific measure of the hamstrings, then the next element of the system goes some way towards redressing the balance. It is necessary to develop **end-of-range, eccentric strength** through single-leg movements. Hamstring injury typically occurs towards the end of the range of movement, and therefore it is only logical to develop strength in the area of greatest risk. Injury is also most likely to occur during eccentric actions and so this specific aspect of strength must be maximised. Part of the appeal of the much-lauded Nordic hamstring curl is that it allows the hamstrings to be eccentrically loaded heavily. In most cases this constitutes what is known as a 'true eccentric', i.e. one in which the force required to control movement is greater than that which the player can produce. Herein lies one of the exercise's potential limitations. For the majority of players, the point of failure on the exercise comes before they have reached the end of range and they have allowed their hamstrings to relax as they drop to the floor. Consequently the majority of the workload is carried out within the inner range, which is not our intended target. This can be addressed by performing the movement on an incline, which reduces the distance of the lever from the fulcrum and therefore reduces the force requirements at this range. However, one interesting study may render this unnecessary. A group of Australian researchers found that despite these limitations, Nordic curls resulted in a shift in the angle of peak torque (i.e. players became stronger towards the end of range).

Another aspect of specificity which must be considered is the context in which the hamstrings are required to produce end of range, eccentric force. We must not forget the fact that hamstring injuries are highly related to central fatigue. The graph in Figure 6.2 illustrates how injury risk increases through the first half of the match,

When is an Eccentric not an Eccentric?

When discussing exercises such as Nordic curls, the definition as 'eccentric' comes from the fact that the muscle is lengthening while under tension. This has remained an uncontroversial view for many years. However, recently evidence is emerging that during Nordic curls and other similar exercises that the muscle fascicles are not lengthening at all throughout the movement. In fact, they may actually be shortening (which would technically make it a concentric movement). It would appear that rather than fascicles lengthening, the movement is accommodated almost entirely in the tendon. This is logical as it allows the muscle to stay closer to optimum length and therefore retain mechanical efficiency. So, if we think in terms of the muscle–tendon unit, we still have an eccentric action. When we talk of eccentric training from here-on-in, it is on this basis rather than a simplistic view of muscle lengthening.

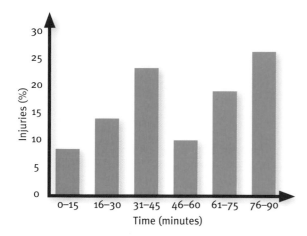

Figure 6.2 Time of Hamstring Strains Sustained
During Match Play
Source: Woods, C, Hawkins, R, Maltby, S, Hulse, M,
Thomas, A, Hodson, A (2004). *The Football
Association Medical Research Programme: an audit
of injuries in professional football* – analysis of
hamstring injuries.

reduces significantly following half-time and then
grows again to its highest level during the final 15
minutes. Therefore we need to develop **eccentric
strength under fatigue**. It has been shown that
eccentric strengthening programmes have
condition-dependent transfer in that if training is
performed free from fatigue, gains are most
evident when the player is fresh. Conversely,
training performed fatigued (such as immediately
after on-pitch sessions) shows a greater transfer to
these conditions. This may provide us with a vital
insight into when we need to schedule these
training bouts into the wider programme.

Finally, we must also seek to develop what I term
functional lengthening. The hamstrings are
required to perform at extreme ranges of
movement, particularly during kicking, when they
are subject to simultaneous knee extension and
hip flexion at high speeds and forces. However,

longer hamstrings per se is not necessarily
something we should seek (excessive stretchers
take note). Acquiring greater range without
strength will merely allow the player to get into
positions of greater vulnerability. Instead, the
player requires strength through range. Therefore
exercises such as good mornings and Romanian
deadlifts (RDLs), which take the muscle through
full range under tension, are extremely useful. As
we have seen already, it may also be the case that
high-force 'eccentric' exercises such as Nordic
curls may also provide the same benefit due to the
lengthening stress placed on the fascicles.

6.5 Muscle Function

Hopefully by now it is not necessary to point out
that simply having a strong muscle is not enough.
It is equally important to have optimal function in
order that the capacity of the muscle is utilised
during activity.

For those players who have suffered previous
injury in this area, there is an additional level of
specificity which must be addressed. Namely, **site
and mechanism of injury specific work**. The most
common site of injury is the myotendinous
junction, due to the large levels of relative stress
across this small cross sectional area. In football
the most common mechanisms of injury are
kicking and sprinting. The site of injury is often left
weakened, thus predisposing the player to
re-injury. This is due to scar-tissue formation,
increases in type III collagen and irregular collagen
orientation. Isokinetic testing and training can be
extremely useful in aiding precision in this regard.
In the hands of a skilled practitioner, aspects of
weakness can be identified within a force trace and
targeted through training. Retraining the player
through the mechanism of injury, be it sprinting or
kicking, is a vital part of the rehab process. Of

course, all players will return to sprinting and kicking as a natural matter of course – this is not the same thing. Well-controlled, carefully progressed doses of this work are required, with good attention to mechanics and perceptions of pain. This is a classic case whereby pain and/or fear of re-injury can inhibit muscle firing and, paradoxically, increase the vulnerability of the hamstrings.

Away from the specific mechanism of injury, it is also prudent to include a variety of **reactivity work** to increase the 'bandwidth of skill' around the hamstrings. The random nature of football dictates that the firing patterns and joint mechanics are constantly changing. Therefore, unlike a closed skill like track sprinting, it is important that the player has great physical literacy to produce an appropriate response to all manner of stimuli. The theory of differential learning dictates that by presenting a wide variety of stimuli the player will acquire skill at a greater rate than if the same specific task is performed repeatedly. As a result, seemingly non-specific exercises such as kicking to focus pads, and a variety of running drills (such as ABC drills) can provide the player with a more robust level of neuromuscular skill.

Sprint running should form part of any hamstring-protection programme as this demands high force and high skill in tandem. However, not all sprinting is created equally. If a player is able to anticipate the motor skills required to perform a task ahead of time, then they have a good chance of executing the skill correctly and with control. An example of this would be sprinting and changing direction between cones. Even when an element of reactivity is introduced, such as responding to a cue from the trainer, the absence of pressure allows the player comfort to perform the skill under control. However, during **opposed running challenges** such as competitive game situations against peers,

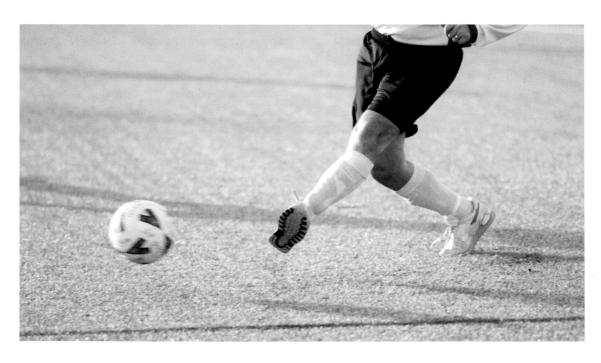

the need to succeed comes first, and control is relegated to second priority. Players returning from injury are particularly vulnerable to this, as a degree of 'rustiness' can make them slightly off the pace and frequently chasing the game, and lacking the control, balance and relaxation which we would seek. For healthy players, this should typically form part of their everyday training stimulus as a matter of course. However, if your monitoring systems allow and a player is particularly vulnerable, it may be prudent to ensure that this dose is optimised and modulated carefully (i.e. make sure they are not doing too much or too little). For rehabbing players, slowly progressing the pace of the task and the level of opponent is important to avoid embarrassing re-injury.

There are few professional clubs who do not perform some form of **isokinetic testing** to assess hamstring function. This is typically done as part of the medical on signing and at the start of pre-season. I think it is fair to say that this can be something of a dark art. On the one hand it represents a highly quantifiable and sensitive measure of hamstring strength, which can be compared to the opposing forces generated by the quadriceps. On the other, the reliability of the results depend much on the motivation of the player and their willingness to give a maximal exertion (often reduced in those who have suffered hamstring injury in the past). This reliability reduces dramatically with higher speeds of movement which presents an issue as these are technically more functional. The interpretation of the results in terms of anomalies within the trace is a high skill and it is far too easy to produce a false hypothesis. Finally, the position of testing is non-functional, and so transfer of results is debateable. That may all sound as if I think isokinetic testing is a waste of time. I don't. Instead

I would simply urge caution and suggest that these limitations are acknowledged. If that sounds obvious, I have witnessed first-hand one of the top clubs in European football take the approach that hamstring health should be determined entirely by an isokinetic test and an MRI scan.

6.6 Stress Modulation

If you have reached this stage of the book it will hopefully not be necessary to explain why the most important element of this multi-faceted system is **training load monitoring and control**. Put simply, if you know what a player's threshold training volumes and intensities look like, if you can measure these with some degree of confidence, and you can intervene when necessary, then you have a pretty good injury prevention system. If you do not have these in place, all the Nordic curls and isokinetic profiles in the world will still leave you with the status of a cross-fingered gambler.

Finally, the significance of **abstract factors** as discussed in the previous chapter are perhaps more relevant to hamstring injury than any other.

6.7 Summary

The scale of the system described above gives some indication of the complexity of hamstring injury prevention. The reality is, even with all of the above elements covered dutifully hamstring injuries will still occur. This is illustrated fantastically in a paper by Dr Peter Bruckner and the Liverpool FC science and medicine team. In their case study of a player suffering numerous hamstring re-injury episodes they paint a very honest picture of how, even with the most attentive and well-qualified team, hamstrings can literally bite you on the rear.

007
specific injury-prevention systems: groin

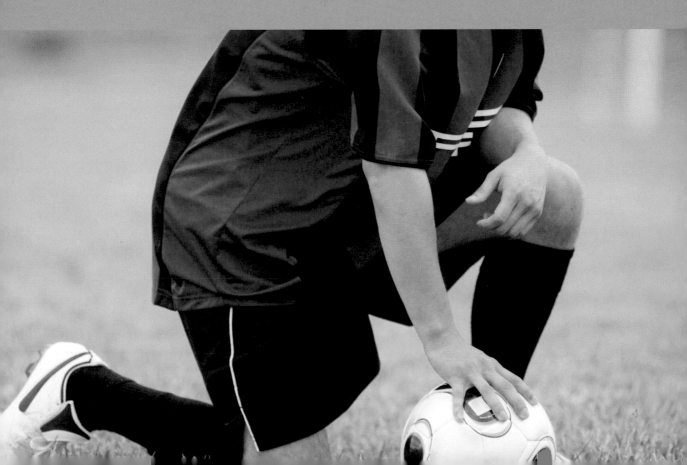

Groin injuries are rapidly becoming 'the new hamstrings' within professional football. As with hamstrings, the prevention and treatment of this injury is rather more complex than most other injury sites.

To be clear from the outset, the term 'groin' refers to the structures at the anterior and medial element of the thigh and into the lower abdomen, including the perineum. It is certainly not simply the adductor muscle group in isolation. Groin pain can arise from a number of sources including adductor strains, hernias, osteitis pubis and labral issues – to name but a few. The diagnosis of these is complex and often unclear. Therefore it is, as ever, vital to work closely with the medical team to gain the greatest possible understanding of the underlying causes when a player complains of groin pain.

Given that groin pain is clearly something of a catch-all term used to describe the symptoms of a number of conditions, an injury-prevention system can only be considered to be painted in broad brushstrokes. However, a number of consistent factors underpin health in this area, namely:

- Abdominal conditioning

- Adductor conditioning

- Hip mobility and pelvic control

These are outlined in Table 7.1 below.

7.1 Trunk Conditioning

Control of the pelvis is key to groin-pain prevention in my experience. Therefore control and conditioning of the musculature of the trunk and hips is vital.

A trunk-conditioning programme should primarily consist of exercises which are what I would term **'iso-dynamic'** in nature. By this I mean that the trunk remains stable through isometric contraction

Table 7.1	Groin Injury-Prevention System		
Trunk Conditioning	**Adductor Conditioning**	**Hip Mobility & Control**	**Testing & Benchmarking**
Emphasis on iso-dynamic work	Muscle capacity (non-functional adduction tasks)	Bespoke work	Adductor-squeeze test
Include adductor-trunk co-contraction & diagonal pattern	Functional capacity	Movement prep warm-ups	Extension control test
'Low-level' work retains constant presence	Functional lengthening		Establish threshold targets
			Establish training dose required

while the limbs are dynamic. This essentially represents the primary function of the trunk musculature – that is, to transfer force effectively during limb movement. This rule applies to performance and injury prevention alike. Generally S&C programmes have moved forward from the days of programmes dominated by sit-ups and crunches, which do not reflect a functional role. However, it is important that while this reflects the primary philosophy we need not be overly dogmatic in this area. The work of leading back specialist Stuart McGill has shown us that there may be room for 'non-functional' exercises due to the very high levels of muscle activation which they elicit.

In my experience, there may be no other aspect of conditioning which better reflects the importance of understanding myofascial slings and the way in which forces are transferred across the body. Forces vectors travel diagonally from the adductors across the abdomen to the contralateral side of the trunk. This gives us several clues as how best to construct exercises that replicate function. **Co-contraction of the abdominals and adductors** is very important. This can be achieved very simply by combining isometric squeezing with trunk training exercises (such as a crunch with a med ball between the knees). Likewise, it is highly desirable to include standing exercises which train the **diagonal patterns** described above. This can include wood-chop type exercises, and proprioceptive neuromuscular facilitation (PNF) patterning work. In this type of movement the force vector is diagonal while the adductors and abdominals function to resist movement making the challenge highly transferrable. The intensity of effort in this type of exercise is generally reduced in a trade-off for the greater neuromuscular specificity.

Finally, **low-level motor control** of the pelvis is absolutely crucial. It is extremely common to find players who are able to perform high-force trunk tasks without loss of form, but lack control in low-force, low-speed tasks. At first this may seem confusing, and it is an easy mistake to assume that if a high-intensity challenge can be met then anything of lower intensity can be achieved also. However, the explanation for this apparent anomaly is that the strategy during the high-intensity task is often to simply 'recruit everything'. However, during the low-level work a good level of fine motor control is required around the pelvis. Therefore not only must this quality be trained, it must be retained. By this I mean one must not simply achieve it and then move on to high-force tasks. They are fundamentally different and should be treated as such within programming. The programming should begin with basic motor education around the pelvis (often delivered by physios), and then transferred into functional tasks such as controlled cycling of the leg to replicate the running action while maintaining a stable trunk and pelvis.

7.2 Adductor Conditioning

The adductors are a muscle group that tend to perform their function in complex movements which require a reasonable amount of skill, and in positions of mechanical disadvantage, i.e. in a position of significant abduction. Consequently there is a large disparity between the forces which can be generated in functional versus non-functional tasks. Therefore there is an enhanced case for the inclusion of both within the training programme.

Much like the hamstrings, high-force, **non-functional conditioning exercises** targeting the adductors can feel uncomfortable, particularly in those who have had injury in this area. Naturally, caution must be taken if discomfort is reported.

However, this work provides a valuable opportunity to optimally strengthen the adductors, which has been demonstrated to reduce injury risk. While it is only based on experience rather than research, I also believe that the nervous system protects the adductors and groin through increased tension in the area. By strengthening the adductors I have found that players are able to gain a greater range of movement. My rationale for this is that they no longer require the 'protection' from being weak in greater ranges. This type of work may be isometric or dynamic, although it is best performed within inner ranges. An imbalance of strength between the adductors and abductors has often been cited as significant risk factor for injury. Therefore the balance of existing strength, as well as the emphasis on each of these elements within the training programme, should be considered when setting strength targets.

Functional strengthening exercises may come in several forms. As we've seen, the adductors are involved in many high-speed, high-force actions which occur towards the end of their range of motion, such as sprinting, cutting, etc. The nature of these tasks means that the timing of muscle firing is equally important to their absolute force-generating capacity. Many of these challenges require a feed-forward neuromuscular response, and a high rate of eccentric force development to resist yielding to ground reaction forces. Well-controlled plyometrics are an obvious exercise choice for developing this type of high-force and high-skill performance. However, there are other functional tasks of lower velocity such as single-leg squat patterns, which are also important and may well act as stepping stones to full-blown high-speed activities.

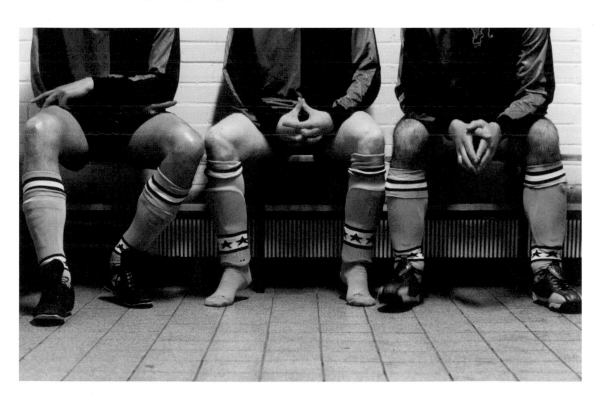

Just as we have seen with the hamstrings, the concept of **functional lengthening** is very important in the adductors. We already know that weak adductors are a high-risk factor for injury, therefore it logically follows that the players who most commonly feel vulnerable in this area are likely to be relatively weak. However, it is infinitely more common to see players performing passive groin stretches than it is to see them performing groin strengthening. Clearly, this serves only give the body greater capacity to move into positions of greater risk as they have gained more range without accompanying strength. Therefore exercises such as sumo deadlifts (or sumo squats), and lunge patterns are vital in taking the adductors through greater range while maintaining active tension.

7.3 Hip Mobility and Control

Far from being a simple case of strengthening a single muscle group such as the adductors, prevention of groin pain and injury demands the optimisation of movement qualities of the myriad factors which affect hip mobility and control.

Factors which are likely to compromise hip function include restriction or asymmetry of medial rotation, tightness through hip flexors, poor control of anterior-posterior pelvic tilt and poor control of lateral pelvic tilt. These issues should have been identified during screening processes, or possibly picked up following medical assessment if pain is reported.

Chronic or more severe cases of restriction or poor control must be addressed through **bespoke programmes** for these players. Ideally this will include bespoke warm-up preparation on top of more in-depth developmental work. It is now pretty much standard practice to include **movement preparation** work as part of the warm-up. This will include squat and lunge patterns, movement drills and mobilisation work. The key here is to ensure that this work is performed to a high standard. This type of activity is inherently low intensity, and the value comes from the quality of movement and attention to detail. It is still commonplace for this to be lacking in squad warm-ups. If this is the case then it is prudent to alert high-risk players to be aware of the exercises which are of particular value to them. Ideally the S&C coach will also be present during the warm-up to assist in the coaching of technical detail and to focus attention of specific players during elements of the session that are highly related to their movement issues.

7.4 Testing and Bench Marking

The **adductor-squeeze test** provides a useful measure of adductor strength and the provocation of pain. The test should be performed in three positions of hip flexion (0, 45 and 90 degrees) with outputs measured via a pressure cuff. Absolute scores may not be a predictor of injury in themselves. However, the establishment of normative values in a given player provides a

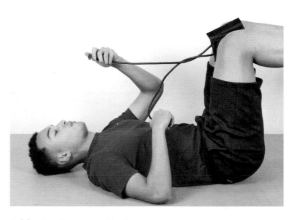

Adductor-Squeeze Test

useful benchmark in players reporting pain or discomfort. Pain or discomfort in the test should be regarded as a highly negative result, and probably more of a concern than a reduction in pressure score. It should be noted that scores can vary somewhat depending on player motivation, fear of pain and tester skill. Therefore it is a useful exercise to understand statistically how much of a change in score is required to represent meaningful change within your specific tester-player group.

The **extension-control test** is an informal gym-based test which is intended to assess lumbo-pelvic isometric control during limb movement. The ability to control extension, and the mechanism through which this is achieved are assessed. The test progresses from a dead bug exercise through to aleknas of various loadings (see below). The primary technical assessment comes from the ability to resist a loss of control at the lumbar spine. This can be assessed through a pressure cuff or simply through manual palpation. Aside from correct technical execution of the movement it is important that the sensation of work comes from the abdominals rather than the lower back. This is considered to represent a mechanical dysfunction as a result of a failure of the low-level trunk musculature.

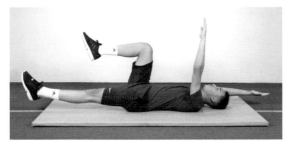

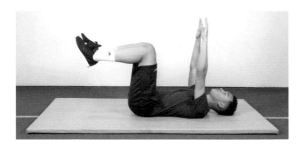

Dead bug

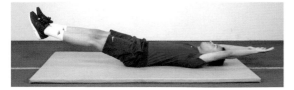

Aleknas

Conditioning for rehabilitation or protection from this type of injury is based on circuit-type sessions, with volume usually based on time rather than repetitions.

7.5 Summary

Groin injury is likely to remain problematic and somewhat mysterious for some time to come. Precise diagnosis and rehabilitation remain elusive in comparison with other injuries. What is clear is that managing the risk factors associated with this type of injury may be the most effective route to minimising the disruption caused by it. The biggest challenge may be achieving the committed and focused adherence to low-level pelvic control in uninjured, pain-free players.

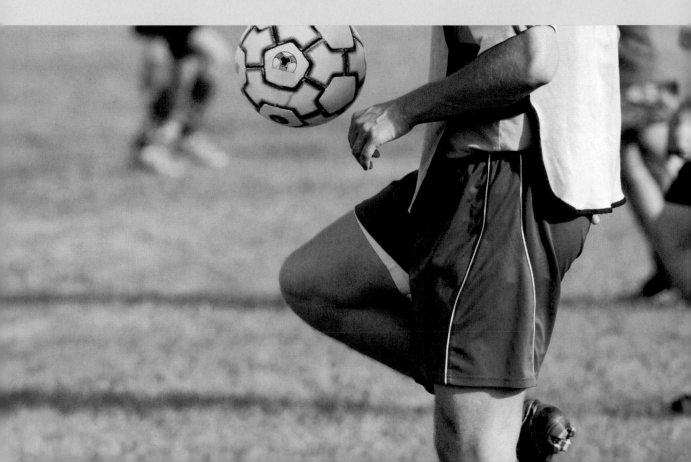

008
specific injury-prevention systems: knee

Unsurprisingly, the knees and ankles are the most commonly injured joints in professional footballers. The knee is of particular concern though, given that the nature of the injury can be catastrophic. Thankfully medical progress means that injuries such as ruptured anterior cruciate ligament (ACL) need no longer be career-ending. That is certainly not to say that they should in any way be taken lightly though. The 6–9 months of rehabilitation represents a significant proportion of a player's playing life, during which they are not developing and improving. Players often come back bearing physical and mental scars, with potential complications such as osteochondral defects.

There are a number of common injuries which may be sustained within the knee joint. Most frequently these include structures such as the ACL, posterior cruciate ligament (PCL), medial and lateral collateral ligaments (MCL and LCL), the meniscus and the patella tendon. This is by no means an exhaustive list, but these are the tissues most likely to bring a player from the pitch to the plinth.

An in-depth discussion around the risk, prevention and treatment of each of these injuries is beyond the scope of this book. However, there are a number of central principles and practices which can help the S&C coach to make a big impact on risk reduction across the squad.

8.1 Strength Qualities

It seems only logical for an S&C coach to think primarily around **strengthening the muscles of the thigh** in order to protect the knee. After all, knees are typically injured when external forces cause them to move into poor positions. In very simple terms, if a player has enough strength to resist these forces then he will avoid injurious positions. If he doesn't, then injury is likely to occur. The full picture is obviously somewhat more complex than this. However, there is no disputing that having the basic strength to resist unwanted movement is a critical factor in protecting a player.

Hopefully it is not necessary to point out to the reader of this book that the methods used to

Table 8.1	Knee Injury-Prevention System	
Strength Qualities	**Motor Control**	**Stress Reduction**
Muscular strength	Stable surface stability	Hip and ankle
Muscular endurance	Unstable surface stability	Running and change of direction mechanics
Rate of force development (RFD)	Balance	Training volume control
Tendon hypertrophy/health	Hip and ankle stability	Consideration given to playing surface
Plyometric ability to resist yielding	Removal of inhibition	

achieve this strength should, in the main, be whole-body, closed-kinetic-chain movements. In simple terms, double- and single-leg squat patterns. These are considered optimal due to the fact that co-contraction of the musculature about the knee is used to control the movement, something which cannot be said of many machine-based exercises. Furthermore, the requirement to control movement helps to transfer strength gains to functional activities both in terms of neuromuscular patterning and a more balanced spread of muscular recruitment. Typically, bilateral patterns are best suited to generating maximal force and developing range-of-movement in the hips and ankles, whereas unilateral patterns shift the emphasis more towards stability.

Allied to muscular strength, local **muscular endurance** is also crucial. A base of strength is vital. However, the ability to produce a true expression of maximal strength is probably lost after the first minute of the game. Thereafter the accumulating fatigue demands that there is some measure of endurance to preserve force capacity during the remaining 89 minutes! As an aside, this concept is often forgotten during movement assessment. The ability to perform a well-balanced squat is important. However the ability to do so *repeatedly* is also important. In terms of programming, endurance should be considered the ability to repeatedly perform to a high level with small bouts of recovery (as this replicates the demands on the knee). This is not to be confused with the ability to work at a low-moderate level for extended periods. In lay terms, 5 sets of 5 reps with short recovery beats endless sets of 12+ squats.

So, in order to retain good control of the knee in the face of potentially damaging forces, the player needs to be able to produce large amounts of counter-force and be able to do so repeatedly. Perhaps the most crucial strength quality, though, is the ability to produce force quickly, i.e. **rate of force development (RFD)**. Whether it be a poorly controlled landing, a blow from an opponent, or an accumulated stress from poor movement patterns, the stressful forces which damage the knee tend to happen quickly. Therefore all the strength in the world is useless if it cannot be called upon in time to prevent negative movements occurring. The natural home for improving RFD is plyometrics (see below). However, this is far from the only way in which it can be developed. Explosive barbell lifts and heavy strength training with an intent to move the bar explosively are both tried-and-tested methods of enhancing RFD. These methods carry the advantage of being highly controllable both in terms of technique and load, and therefore the skilled practitioner will use a blend of plyometrics and strength training to achieve the goal of enhanced RFD depending on, among other things, the specific make-up of the player.

The case for including pre-emptive **tendon strengthening** work is made during Chapter 4. Naturally the knee is a primary site for such work. In the longer term, every effort should be made to optimise mechanics locally and globally in order to reduce the load burden on the patella tendon. However, it is also prudent to maximise tendon health and strength as an insurance policy. In players reporting knee pain there can be a paradoxical balancing act in terms of placing stress on the patella tendon to promote health (which may cause discomfort) and provoking excessive pain.

On a very simplistic level, strength training is primarily about adapting structures, whereas **plyometric training** is about acquiring skill (although of course both include elements of each). As we have already mentioned, plyometrics have the potential to improve RFD. This can be done in highly specific tasks and therefore transfer to performance is likely to be robust. It is important that we distinguish between high-speed, large-impact plyometrics designed for power development and tasks intended to improve stability. The speed of many high-intensity plyos can mask a lack of stability and leave the coach with a false impression of control. Therefore it is important to focus on work which replicates the functional challenges experienced in game play, targets identified movement weaknesses, and exposes any lack of control.

8.2 Motor Control

As we have already touched upon, control of the knee is critical in order to protect it from damaging impacts and forces. The debate surrounding unstable versus stable training has already been highlighted in Chapter 4.

To reiterate, my personal view is that the bulk of stability work should be conducted on a **stable surface**. This goes beyond the obvious flippant defence that football is not played on a wobble board, BOSU or Swiss ball. Primarily I feel that the need for the body to achieve stability through a feed-forward mechanism is crucial. However, I have seen practitioners who are highly experienced in rehab get excellent results through **unstable surface training**. What is lost in motor specificity may be compensated for by an increase in muscle activity. Ultimately I do not believe there is a categorical right or wrong way to develop stability. However, whichever way you structure this type of work I would urge you to have a coherent system, based on a logical thought process, which you can review and refine to build up your own evidence-based system.

To many, **balance** and stability are the same thing … however, these people are wrong! Stability refers to our ability to retain movement control in the face of opposition – such as controlling a landing, etc. Balance refers to our ability to maintain posture in the absence of opposition, although potentially through a compromised position, such as on one leg. Because these represent distinct motor skills, which can be proven by seeing how players commonly exhibit one but not the other, then they must be trained as such. Balance training in uninjured players can be a hard sell as it can seem boring, and therefore engagement and quality can be hard to attain. Therefore it is most effectively incorporated into warm-ups and 'disguised' into other activities which hold the attention. When planned skilfully, these activities can be constructed in a way which demand good form and control (i.e. coaching by stealth).

Gross movement errors, such as a large valgus collapse at the knee, are often the symptom of a problem lying elsewhere in the kinetic chain. The biggest villains of the peace in this regard are **ankle and hip stability**. This is hardly a revelation, as physios and S&C coaches alike are generally aware of the influence of the hip and ankle in knee stability. However, remedying the problem effectively is something far fewer practitioners achieve. The skill lies firstly in the ability to correctly diagnose where in the isolated-functional continuum the motor control deficit lies. The coach must then progressively develop this control, in tandem with strength qualities, to a point where the improvements are evident and robust in the field of play. Often this requires the combined skill sets of the therapist and the S&C coach to turn low-level motor re-education into gross neuromuscular patterns. With regard to hip stability, key questions to consider when evaluating training targets include: is the player able to recruit the gluteals in the correct kinetic sequence; are they able to produce this skill during high-speed, high-force, complex tasks; are they able to produce large amounts of force rapidly; and do they have the endurance capacity to do all of the above repeatedly? With regard to the ankles, the key training considerations lie in the nature of the stability challenge which is placed on the foot and ankle. Task specificity is key, as is the nature of the surface on which they land (as we have already discussed). The foot itself also merits evaluation, as poor control of the foot obviously has implications at the ankle. A comparison of exercise performance with and without shoes can often be very insightful in this regard.

Previous knee injury can often lead to an **inhibition of the quadriceps**. This can result in a terrible paradox whereby the protective inhibition of the muscles around the knee result in the joint moving into more stressful positions, and subsequently suffering further damage. For example, when the foot is planted to land, change direction, etc., the goal is to achieve mechanical stability and avoid yielding at the knee (within limits as high levels of stiffness will increase stress on tendons). However, when inhibition is present, the degree of yield is naturally greater and so the knee travels further over the toes, increasing the anterior stress. The key to breaking free from this vicious cycle is to gently introduce low-level stress prior to training and playing. By starting with low-force impacts and building through a graded increase over 5–10 minutes it is possible to significantly reduce inhibition. For many years I have used a basic plyometric protocol to move from small, double-footed rebound jumps on a soft surface to single-leg rebounding on a firm surface. The contrast can be stark with players commonly moving from heavy, long contacts with lots of muscular effort, to sharp quick contacts with good use of tendon elasticity. This then gives the player the opportunity to train effectively and break out from the inhibition-damage cycle.

8.3 Stress Reduction

Just as poor motor control can result in undue stress on the knee, so can poor gross-movement patterns and technique.

If we begin with basic function movement, **mobility of the hips and ankles** is just as key as stability in these joints. These factors can be dissected via a form of movement screen, even if it is as simple as the ability to perform a basic squat pattern. Any S&C coach who has worked with more than a handful of players will know that the constraints of modern living mean that tight ankles and hips are common issues across athletes in the vast majority of sports. A squat pattern may not be a shape you typically see on a football pitch, but it is certainly one which may help keep you on one. It is for this reason that I would far rather see a player able to perform a good, deep squat with low load, than a moderate-depth squat with a bit more weight. It should be pointed out that it has consistently been demonstrated that not only is a deep squat entirely safe in terms of knee health, it is actually a more stable position than a 90° squat.

Moving on from generic functional movements it is important to look at technique in highly specific movements such as **running, decelerating and changing direction**. Accepting that these skills are underpinned by general movement qualities such as squat patterns, it is necessary to see what happens when a player combines all the factors which determine movement to produce their end result. We could talk for hours on this topic and the combinations of movement challenges and physical attributes which produce an almost endless number of possibilities. However, the critical point with regard to knee health is to achieve positions which allow the hips to produce and reduce force and spread the load, to reduce the burden on the knee. I am always happy to defer to the wisdom of Frans Bosch on such matters, who talks about the importance of the 'plant from above'. This refers to the fact that force is directed downward and in the direction you wish to travel.

It may sound flippant to suggest that the easiest way to reduce stress to the knees is to reduce the amount of training performed. However, **training volume control** is absolutely vital. The amount of stress sustained by a given player's knees will vary tremendously across a squad. All the factors which we have already discussed, such as motor control, technical movement, as well as the nature of their game (i.e. distances covered, number of decelerations, etc.) will affect the accumulated stress. What's more, the ability to tolerate this stress will also vary between players. Therefore it is fundamental to develop a clear picture of acceptable volumes and how to manipulate them, as well as movement patterns and training sessions, which are likely to impact on a player.

Injury prevention is very much a case of risk management rather than elimination. Therefore it is important to be cognisant of all the major factors which contribute to risk and their relative impact. The influence of the **playing surface** is one which must be considered given the varied nature of surfaces in an outdoor sport. Particularly in the UK, fairly significant changes can occur to a playing surface over a short period of time. It is a common occurrence for this to happen at a rate far greater than that to which the body can adapt, and therefore players are exposed to unfamiliar

conditions, and in turn, increased risk. Both empirically and within the literature it would appear that the risk of muscular injuries is greatest during soft ground conditions, while tendon injuries are the greatest risk when the ground is hard. The key to utilising this information is to gain an understanding of the implications for training. If a player is being closely managed as an injury risk and prescribed a particular volume, what is the magnitude of the effect of a change in the playing surface? This is not an easy question to answer, although good use of longitudinal injury data (along with playing surface information) can go a long way to providing an answer.

8.4 Summary

While far from an easy task, the minimisation of knee injuries seems to represent a very tangible goal for the S&C coach. Achieving the requisite strength qualities should be considered a bare minimum which, when backed-up with good motor control programmes and movement mechanics, can have a big impact on players' short- and long-term health.

Finally, the increased incidence of ACL injury in female players is clearly a key consideration for this population. Despite a widespread and longstanding awareness of this issue, it remains a significant problem. Coaches should, however, be encouraged that although the injury rate remains elevated, interventions targeting strength and motor control have been shown to significantly reduce ACL injury rates in female players.

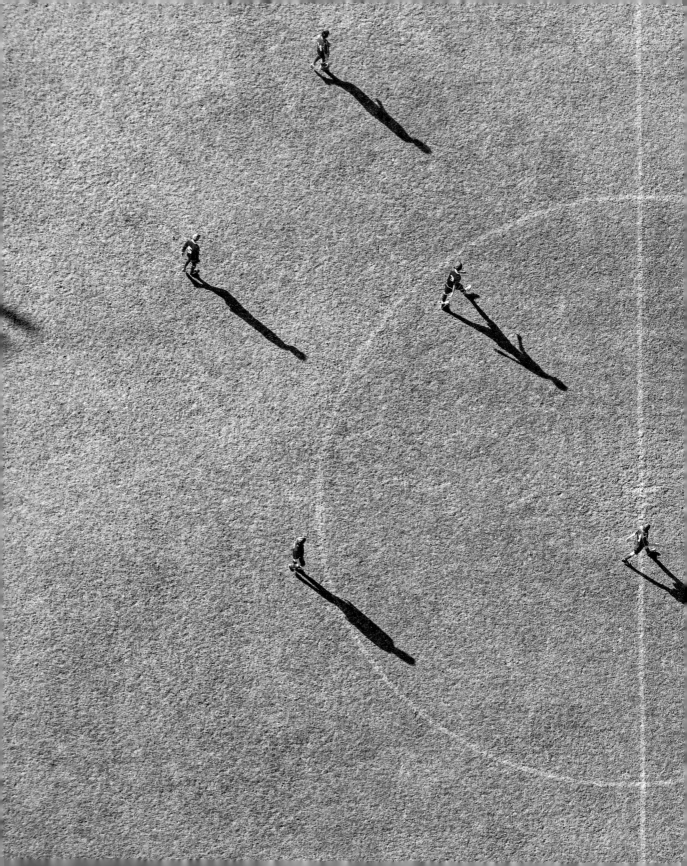

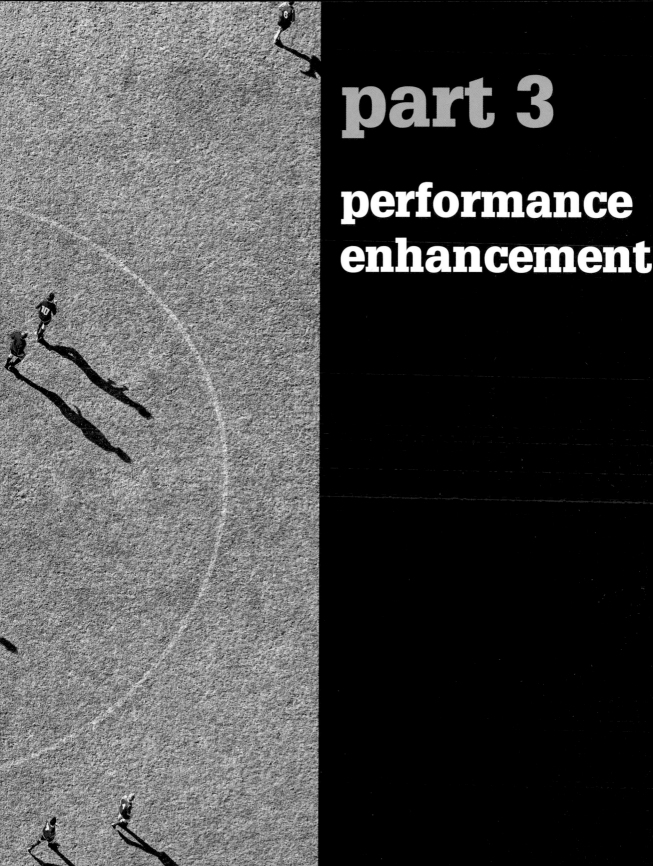

part 3

performance enhancement

009
fundamental principles of performance enhancement

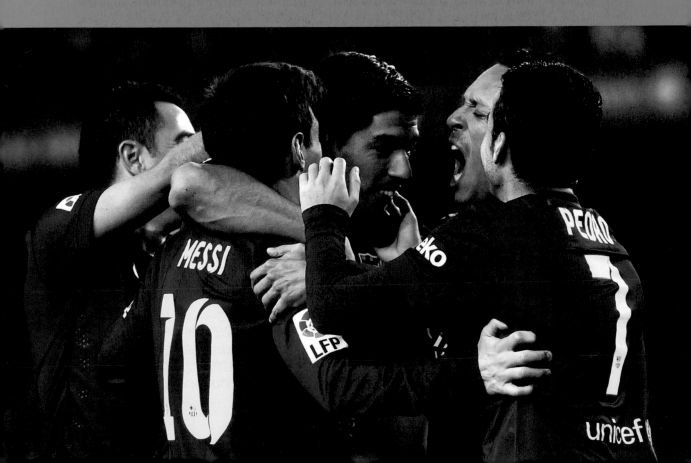

Up to this point our focus has largely been on the prevention of injury. However, it is the nature of the S&C coach to always look for ways to enhance performance as well.

In terms of an underpinning philosophy of performance enhancement we can revisit the performance model described in Chapter 2. To be precise, our efforts are aimed at developing **'Athletic ability to support specific role requirements'**. This goal has been worded very carefully. It is not a fruitful approach to simply develop athletic qualities ad nauseam. Nor is it sufficient to base training goals solely on a player's position. Instead, we need to understand what their role is within the team, which qualities they draw upon to be successful in this role, and which qualities need developing to minimise their weaknesses. This alone presents a philosophical dilemma – do you target the strength or the weakness? (Personally I would always focus on the weakness as it represents the greatest potential for gains. Interestingly, on a macro level it has been demonstrated that improving the weakest player is much more impactful that improving the best player.)

Many still take the generic view that making a player faster, higher, stronger will automatically lead to them being a better player. But have they considered the fact that the way in which they play the games means the majority of players don't actually reach their top running speed at any point during a game? This does not necessarily mean that speed is not worth developing, as we will explore later on. Instead it simply illustrates that a little more thought is required before assuming that enhancing a physical quality will also mean enhancement of match performance.

9.1 Identifying Areas of Impact

There are a number of ways to skin this particular cat. In reality the likelihood is that the system you use will be the one which you inherit.

'Barcelona' model

During the late 1990s, Louis van Gaal, Frans Hoek and Lluis Lainz outlined a performance model based system at FC Barcelona which continues to influence the approach of many top European clubs today. This model begins with the philosophy of the club, which leads into the vision that they wish to achieve. This vision is underpinned by principles of how football matches will be won. For example, *'When transitioning from losing to winning the ball, the most important objective is that the opponent is not yet organised positionally to create chances of scoring a goal as quickly as possible.'*

This is taken into great depth and expanded into tactical formations based on potential situations within a game relating to the score, time remaining, etc. Now that this blueprint for the team as a whole has been clearly defined, they are able to start to determine the requirements for its constituent parts (i.e. the players). Again, this is done in impressive depth and includes a breakdown of the technical, tactical and even psychological requirements of a player in each position. An example of the physical requirements of the number 3 and 4 players (central defenders) is given below:

- Speed in short, medium and long distance
- Power of shot and pass
- Power of heading and power of jump height
- Power of duel
- Agility

Source: van Gaal, L., et al. (2012), *Barcelona Philosophy*.

If I were to be ultra-critical, the only thing missing from this model as it is presented is objective measures of each of these qualities. For example, short speed as represented by 0–5m sprint time and a classification of what is good, poor and average. Hopefully you can see that armed with this type of specific information as to what the coaches need from a player is hugely empowering for an S&C coach. It allows work to be directed in a precise and deliberate manner, with the confidence that it is genuinely performance impacting. It even helps to prioritise work. If a player matches the technical, tactical and psychological metrics required but falls short physically, then the priority of time with the S&C

coach increases dramatically. This is clearly more power to our arm.

Regrettably, the vast majority of professional football does not currently work in such an enlightened and pioneering manner, although hopefully this represents the direction of travel which others will follow. In the meantime we face compromise. However, the point of pioneers is they make the path for those behind them far easier to traverse. With this excellent model as an example and the powerful reputation of Barcelona to enforce the point, I would urge all those involved in science and medicine in football to influence upward and outward through

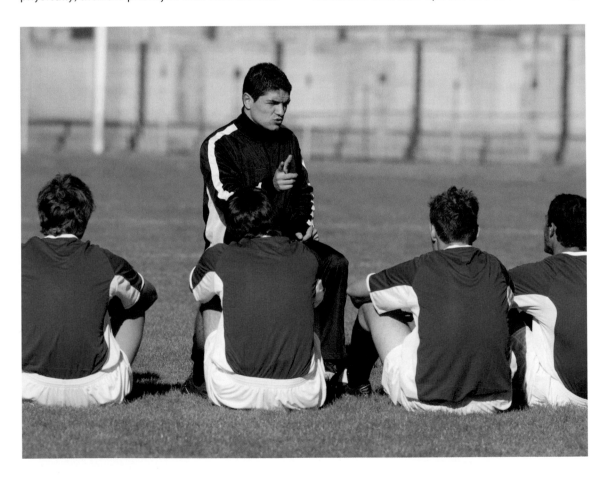

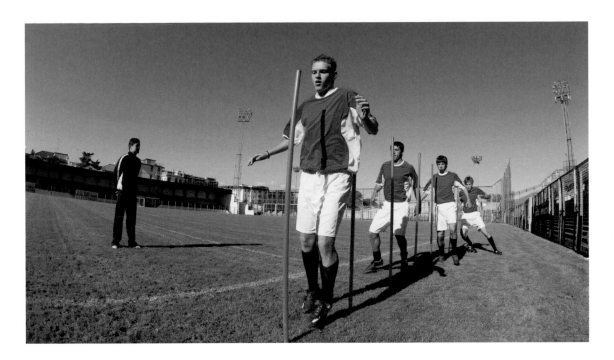

their clubs to promote a shift towards this performance approach.

Performance-Analysis Model

Performance analysis in football now comes in many forms. Most professional clubs now employ a team of in-house PAs. The sports science department often collects movement data through GPS and accelerometer technology. All this comes on top of the array of match analysis companies such as Opta and Prozone, who scrutinise every possible metric within the game in search of greater levels of insight.

All of this data gives us a very quantifiable picture of what a player looks like, and how they compare with their peers. It can tell us which elements of the game make them effective and where their vulnerabilities lie. In theory this could be used as a solitary source of guidance as to how best to develop a player. Of course I would not advocate a

sports science department working In isolation in this way. Instead it should be done in collaboration with coaches and the players themselves. PA can certainly serve as a useful check to ensure that coaching interventions are directed appropriately. I have seen on many occasions how a received wisdom can quickly become treated as a solid fact when, in fact, it carries little real validity. For example, 'Player x needs more acceleration, he always gets done for pace with a ball over the top'. It would not be uncommon if it turned out that this has only happened twice but it caught someone's eye and became a fact – ignoring the plethora of times the same player coped in an identical situation. Just as PA can disprove a myth, it can also be useful for generating new information, giving clues as to where impact can be made. Finally, the mass of readily available video and analysis software now means that once an issue has been identified, such as the ability to cut to the right, it is possible to draw on lots of real-life examples and diagnose the underlying cause. This is a critical part of the process.

Figure 9.1 illustrates a process of both information gathering and validation which uses PA to not only ensure that performance-enhancement interventions are appropriately targeted, but also to provide information to assist in the diagnosis of underlying issues and the subsequent solutions.

The 'Intuitive' Model

In truth this is not a model as there is no formal structure. However, it represents the system that is probably most widely used in professional football.

The essence of this approach is that it is based on assumption. If a player asks to work on an element of their game, there is an assumption that he has selected the most impactful aspect. This of course has many flaws, as players often prefer to work on the things they enjoy. Perceived weaknesses may be skewed by a number of psychological factors, particularly when they relate to body composition and strength. Further assumption is relied upon when the S&C coach makes a diagnosis as to how best to address the issue. For example, it may be tempting to leap to explosive power development to improve acceleration, when in fact the player is primarily limited by their ability to read the game. Finally, this way of working tends to promote practitioners working in silos rather than in an inter-disciplinary manner to solve problems more holistically.

Clearly then, in comparison with the well-planned, strategic joined-up approaches outlined above, this method has a number of weaknesses. However, it is not all bad. If coaches and players are approaching you to work on performance then you have clearly gained their trust. It is often the case

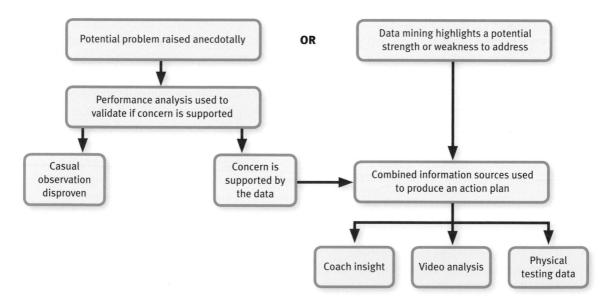

Figure 9.1 Performance-Analysis Performance-Enhancement Model

10.1 The Need for Speed

The most compelling case for S&C to enhance performance comes from the capacity to improve locomotive abilities. This includes acceleration, deceleration, maximum speed and the various subcategories of change of direction (CoD).

In the previous chapter the point was made that many players do not come anywhere near their maximum speed during match play. This was intended to demonstrate that getting quicker will not necessarily directly translate to enhanced performance. However, when we dig slightly deeper there is more to be gained from improving speed capacity than simply beating the opponent to the ball in all-out races.

The excellent applied sports scientist, Martin Buchheit, has illustrated very clearly how maximal sprint speed influences the physiology of working at slower speeds. Figure 10.1 below shows how two players who run at similar speeds at VO_{2max} may be working at different percentages of their anaerobic speed reserve (ASR). Essentially this means that player B has their foot on the gas to a much lesser extent than player A, without having better aerobic fitness. Personally I have seen a very real example of this with a Premier League player who was sorely lacking in speed. His position did not demand that he run expansive distances or hit great speeds. However, the fact that he was constantly operating so close to his relatively low maximum speed made him vulnerable to injury and burn-out. There is no doubt in my mind that improving this player's top speed, and therefore speed reserve, would have a big impact on his game, even though he would never actually use it.

In addition to the benefits of a large ASR, there are multiple benefits to having good running technique. Of course, it is obvious that by improving technique we can improve our maximum speed, ability to accelerate, decelerate and CoD. Let's think about exactly what technique means though. Another way of saying technique could be our mechanical expression of force. If we improve this then, yes we can potentially raise our maximum, but gains are not limited to top-end efforts. By improving how we express force we can also move more efficiently. As we have already discussed, this economy of movement may be more important than top speed for many players. Furthermore, a system which has good mechanical efficiency also endures less mechanical stress. Consequently, improving running technique can have big implications for reducing injury risk (we will discuss some of the specifics of this later on).

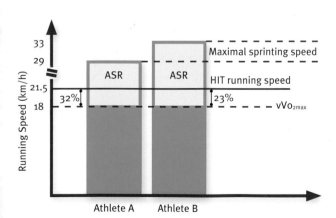

Figure 10.1 Importance of Anaerobic Speed Reserve Source: Buchheit, M. and Laursen, B. (2013). 'High Intensity Interval Training, Solutions to the Programming Puzzle', *Sports Med* (43).

10.2 Diagnosing the Problem

Debating the best approach for enhancing locomotive abilities is not a simple task. Essentially the coach must evaluate the technique and mechanics of a player as well as their physical qualities to establish where the greatest opportunities for gains lie. Increasing strength and power may be an inefficient approach if poor mechanics in running and CoD are wasteful or do not allow for gains to be expressed. Conversely, changing mechanics will yield little or no gain if the player does not have the raw capability to produce force.

One novel method of determining whether the greatest deficit lies in technique or physical qualities can be drawn from a comparison of jump and sprint performance. The strong relationship between explosive power during jumping and sprint speed is well established. Both within the literature and from my own data gathering, correlations of around 0.7–0.8 can be seen between elements of jump performance and sprint metrics. Typically this information has been used to support the case for explosive gym training towards improving game speed. However, there may be a more creative opportunity to gain insight into a player's make-up.

Figure 10.2 illustrates typical data which can be gathered by comparing countermovement jump (CMJ) height and 30m sprint times. The trendline through the graph represents the typical sprint–jump relationship. While the correlation isn't perfect (0.7 in this example), it does give us some indication as to how effectively a player is utilising their explosive power to produce speed during sprinting. If the player sits close to this line then it suggests that there is a reasonable equilibrium between technique and physical ability (or at least in comparison to the rest of the group). However, a player sitting significantly above the line may be considered somewhat slower than would be expected given their jumping ability. This may lead to suspicion that their expression of force

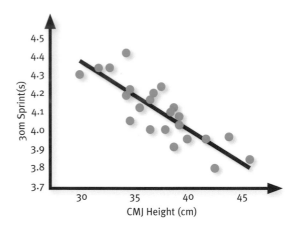

Figure 10.2 The Relationship Between 30m Sprint and Jumping Ability
Source: Jarvis case-study data

(i.e. technique) is not particularly effective. On the other hand, a player sitting below the line is faster than our equation would predict, and thus we may draw the conclusion that they have above average technique and ability to use their existing qualities. So, the first player may benefit most from technical work, whereas the second may be best directed towards improving strength qualities.

Now, before we go too far with this concept I should point out that there are a number of weaknesses to the theory. Firstly, we must not forget that the act of jumping requires a degree of skill and technique, and therefore cannot be considered a pure measure of physical qualities. Secondly, the correlation is not perfect, which leaves some room for error. This error can be reduced by being more specific with the components of strength and running assessed. Correlations as high as 0.86 have been found between starting speed (first 2.5m) and peak force during jumping. The same study also showed a correlation of 0.8 between maximal sprinting speed and the force applied at 100m during jumping.

For all these concerns, there is still a useful insight to be gained through this simple analysis – we just cannot treat it as an absolute truth. Rather, it simply acts as another piece of the puzzle and assists our ability to make objective decisions regarding the best method to enhance a player's performance. Furthermore, this system may be of value when assessing the potential of a player to enhance their sprinting abilities. This may be a youth player whom the club's coaches need to make a decision on, or even a prospective transfer coming for a medical assessment. Firstly, it is of value to be able to gauge the trainability of the player (i.e. do their abilities suggest they could be quicker?). Secondly, the predictive trendline may give a crucial guide as to how much quicker the player could be. This is vital in terms of managing the expectations of coaches. As we know, speed is strongly linked to genetics. It is often said that sprinters are born, not made. There have been countless examples of talented players who aren't quite quick enough, leading the coach to constantly ask the S&C coach if they can make them quicker. The answer should generally be, 'yes, but only a bit'. This system may allow a more objective and quantifiable answer.

10.3 Running Technique

If we wish to assess and potentially train running technique then we need a clear technical model to work from. In my experience there are very few people in the game historically who have clearly defined their running model. The traditional approach was for coaches to defer all running expertise to sprint coaches. This typically meant that the players whose choice of parent dictated that they would be type-I muscle-fibre dominant

were sent off to spend several weeks over the summer with a sprints coach. This would be done with a view to some kind of miracle transformation from tortoise to hare. Aside from the physiological challenge, this was generally limited by a fixed view of sprint mechanics and coaching methods which do not translate well to a different population. The situation may have moved on somewhat, as there are some more enlightened sprints coaches and S&C coaches now have some level of knowledge in this area. However, there are still very few genuine specialists with a proven track record of making meaningful changes in players.

To move forward, we need to clearly define what we are trying to build, and establish how well a player needs to be able to run for us to be satisfied that efforts are best directed elsewhere. It is probably fair to say that most players do not run particularly well. This is only to be expected as it is an acquired skill which must be taught if it is to be executed to a high level. That said, a number of players can move pretty quickly and so, for all the apparent technical deficiencies, they are obviously doing a number of things right. Most would agree that the technical proficiency demonstrated by Olympic sprinters is not required (or even appropriate). So where do we draw the line in the sand?

I believe that the answer lies in the critical positions theory. Essentially this means that there are a number of key positions which must be achieved within a sports skill in order to be effective. As long as the technique allows these to be reached, the rest, for the most part, is academic. An extreme example of this comes from the golfer, Jim Furyk. Furyk was known for his highly unorthodox swing which has been described as looking like 'a one-armed golfer trying to hit a ball with an axe in a phone box'. Despite apparently drifting so far from the technical model, Furyk was able to remain among the most successful golfers on the tour throughout his career. The reason for this is that he hit the critical positions, such as the point at which the club face meets the ball, correctly. There are many similar examples in football with players who on the surface appear to run poorly, but are actually quite effective. The opposite can also be true. This simply highlights the need for a well-considered model to measure against.

10.4 Key Components of Good Running

The specific mechanics required are obviously dependent on the task, i.e. acceleration versus top speed versus CoD, etc. However, the components of technique which we are concerned with do not change.

Arguably the single most important element of running technique is **posture**. As Bosch and Klomp state, '...movement in the trunk and pelvis play an important and frequently underestimated role during running'. While the eye of many coaches is immediately drawn to the limbs, technical deficiencies here are often merely the symptom of a lack of control earlier in the kinetic chain. An interesting study carried out by skill-acquisition experts, including Oliver Logan at the English Institute of Sport, tracked the visual gaze of elite sprints coaches versus novice S&C coaches. They found that the eye of the sprints coach was predominantly focused on the hips and pelvis, whereas the novice coaches looked at many more areas and spent more time on distal segments such as the ankles. If the pelvis is stable and properly aligned then the limbs can move appropriately, efficiently and effectively. That is certainly not to say that the pelvis should be fixed and rigid – stability does not mean a total absence of movement. The pelvis should be free to rotate through all three planes of movement.

Defining how much movement is acceptable is a near impossible question to answer as it very much depends. It is common for medics to observe a running action and speak of 'excessive' movement in the pelvis. But how do we know it is excessive? Perhaps it is more useful to think in terms of the degree and mechanism of control. For example, a player may run with very little movement through anterior-posterior pelvic tilt. However, if this stability is achieved through jamming the pelvis into a fixed anterior tilt at the end of range, there are severe implications for spinal health and other injuries. A pattern which uses good neuromuscular control to stay within a bandwidth of movement is far preferable to fixing using the joint. Equally, movement which a player does not have good control over is likely to have implications further down the kinetic chain (i.e. reduced force output and/or compensatory movement patterns).

The posture in the trunk obviously begins with the standing posture of the player. If this is poor then it is inevitable that the same will be true during running. The desired running posture is frequently described as 'running tall' with 'high hips'. This is often misinterpreted within football and is met with the argument that they should not run like sprinters. However, the posture is more appropriately considered in relation to the rest of the body rather than the ground. The images on page 95 illustrate how good posture does not automatically mean tall, erect running.

There can be little argument over the consideration of **foot placement** as a key component of all forms of running. After all, our only opportunity to produce, reduce or redirect force is through contact

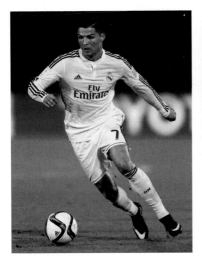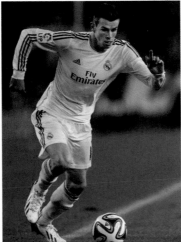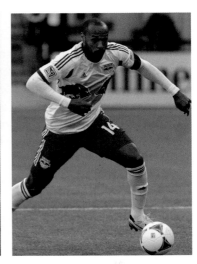

Figure 10.3 Christiano Ronaldo, Gareth Bale and Thierry Henry

Table 10.1	Acceleration vs. High-Speed Running
ACCELERATION	**HIGH SPEED**
Foot is placed to direct force behind the knee and in front of the hip (negative shin angle).	Foot placed under centre of mass projection.
Knee strongly bent at the start of first few strides to use extension power of the quads. This gradually decreases.	Knee and hip flexion will be matched at contact, large flexion at each means 'sitting down'. This may result in failure to generate thrust with the hamstrings.
The ankle should be strongly dorsi-flexed with a large amount of tension.	Stable unmoving ankle required.
Full triple extension at toe off.	Incomplete triple extension at toe off.
Active hip flexion at toe off.	Active hip flexion at toe off.
Foot placement will be somewhat externally rotated which may help push the free hip lower or exert more force through tighter adductors, etc. – it is of little use trying to change this.	Knees side-by-side at foot placement.
Body angle of approx. 45° on first step, gradually rising.	
Swing leg is kept low for first few strides to minimise time between ground contacts.	

Adapted from: Bosch & Klomp (2005)

with the ground. The position of the foot in relation to the rest of the body will have a profound effect on our ability to do so. The horizontal distance of the foot placement from the hips is determined by the desired outcome. If the goal is to continue to move at the same or greater speed without a change in direction the distance should be minimal, i.e. under the hips, to avoid braking impulse. In a change of direction the distance increases with the

severity of change. In rapid deceleration the distance should be maximised. Table 10.1 below summarises some of the other key differences in the requirements of accelerations and high-speed running.

In my experience of having watched and worked with many footballers, the biggest impact which can be had over their gross technique is to effect a shift **from rear-side to front-side mechanics**. These are terms first used by the running biomechanist, Ralph Mann. They refer to the proportion of the gait cycle which occurs to the rear or the front of the midline of the body. In order to run quickly it is necessary to direct downward vertical force into the ground. The movement of the leg from toe off through the swing phase plays a huge role in determining the mechanical opportunity to do so. When running with front-side dominant mechanics, the hip and knee of the swing leg flex simultaneously. This results in a 'stepping over the knee' type action, with the thigh being lifted and the player in a position to then powerfully generate downward thrust. However, the rear-side pattern which is commonly observed sees the knee flex at toe off with a greatly delayed flexing of the hips. Consequently there is what is known as a 'pendulum swing', which sees the back leg trailing behind the body with the foot floating up high.

An easy way to observe these actions is the direction of travel of the foot during the swing phase. In rear-side running the foot moves from high to low, whereas the opposite is true of front-side running. Critically the end position, as shown above, means that when the hip has been flexed actively and early, the player can use the hips to drive down hard towards the ground. If not, not only is force generation compromised

A Word about the Arms

For some reason I have never fully understood, TV punditry of athletics seems to exclusively review performances in sprint races with footage of the athletes from the waist upward. As a consequence, many people tend to associate good sprint technique as disproportionately being about the arm action.

It is not true that the arms help to drive a player forward. Instead, the chief role of the arm action is to generate downward thrust and control rotation. In his research, Ralph Mann found no association between horizontal speed and either arm position or velocity. It may be going too far to suggest that we ignore the action of the arms altogether. However, the arms themselves are often merely a symptom of another problem, for example, a lack of rotational control of the trunk, or an excessive pendulum swing causing an over-rotation.

The take-home message is that before leaping in with arm-action drills, first deal with postural control and an effective gait cycle. The chances are that if you do this effectively, the problem will have taken care of itself.

(meaning slower or less efficient running) but the action becomes more of a pull than a push. It is important to realise that this does not just apply to sprinting. Of course, during jogging and running the thigh does not need to be lifted as high as during sprints. However, we should still be looking for a smaller version of the same shape. I believe that a lot of players accumulate undue fatigue in the hamstrings due to this poor running action. It causes them to accumulate large volumes of work as a concentric hip extensor.

It is my firm view that shifting running bias towards front side is the single most impactful way to positively affect the majority of footballers. In addition to the specific rationale outlined above, there are often knock-on implications for posture, foot placement and a balance of relaxation and mechanical stiffness.

10.5 Assessing Running Technique

In order to evaluate the potential for technical change to enhance speed in a player, it is necessary to make some form of structured assessment of their current technique. It is important that this is done in an objective, quantifiable manner. It is easy for S&C coaches and others to fall into the habit of criticising a player's technique and picking out all of the faults. Apart from not being particularly constructive, this is also not very informative. Instead we need a system which is repeatable between individuals and is proven to assess the components of running technique which really matter, rather than those which catch the eye.

It is crucial to capture good-quality footage of the player running. This not only gives us the opportunity to closely evaluate the positions they

Football-Specific Running Technique

There are numerous times within a game when it is necessary to run in a relatively straight line and without a ball. Therefore the ability to simply run in the most effective way possible is required.

However, there are also occasions such as dribbling at speed, or when there may be a need to rapidly change direction when running mechanics need to be altered. The higher the cadence of stride, the more frequently the player will have an opportunity to alter their path or take a touch on the ball.

Ronaldo is often cited as having a very effective running style, as his cadence is often very high, meaning that he stays in touch with the ball very effectively. However, this may not be a great model to draw on. It is only due to exceptional physical qualities that he is able to perform in this way. Running with such an extreme stride length–frequency requires extreme speed capabilities. If the average player attempted to run in this way, opponents would most likely jog past them!

In reality, Ronaldo just serves as an extreme example of how the generic technical model can be adapted to accommodate football skill. Critically, it is still the same pattern that we are trying to promote but to a lesser extent, i.e. we still want front-side mechanics and an active knee drive, we simply change the parameters.

reach in clear detail, but also serves as a record for comparison after any training interventions. Nowadays the ability to capture good-quality footage, slow it down and freeze frames is available to pretty much all of us.

As we have already discussed, the ability to hit critical positions is quite possibly the best way of evaluating the effectiveness of a player's technique. The work of the leading biomechanists in running suggests that these positions are Stance, Toe Off and the front and rear portions of the Swing Phase. The key elements of these aspects are described in Table 10.1. Table 10.2 below gives an example of a player graded against the criteria of each of these positions. The illustrations provide an example of a player being assessed at each of the positions, with comments on the performance given adjacent. To illustrate how this could be quantified for comparison each element has been given a rating between 0 and 2. Good technical execution scores 2, adequate but room for improvement scores 1 point, and poor technique scores 0.

10.6 The Mechanics of Changing Direction

It is important to begin with an acceptance that CoD, or agility, is as much a cognitive task as it is a physical one. Initially this comes from the ability to recognise a stimulus. This may be from an opponent, a teammate, or both. Top players are often defined by their ability to do so. This is perhaps illustrated at its best by the well-documented study carried out by the University of Calgary, focusing on Ronaldo. They illustrated how he was able to accurately determine the flight and speed of a cross simply from watching a player's hips. Similarly, while a lower-level player in a one-on-one focused mainly on the ball, Ronaldo's visual gaze focused heavily on the opposition player's body (largely hips and balance), and followed a very consistent pattern. This is just one example of what is consistently seen when elite and novice players are compared.

Once the player has read the stimuli available to them they can execute the second phase: decision making. These two first components often

Table 10.2	Example Evaluation of Acceleration Critical Positions		
Stance	**Toe off**	**Swing phase (rear)**	**Swing phase (front)**

Table 10.2	Example Evaluation of Acceleration Critical Positions (cont.)	
	Comments	**Rating**
Stance phase:		
Correctly sequenced triple extension throughout (hip to knee to ankle)	Adequate	1
Continual hip flexion of swing leg throughout all of stance	Hip flexion ends early (2–3 frames prior to toe off)	1
At the point of full hip flexion the knee angle will be ($\leftarrow\cdots$) 90°	Currently approx. 109°	1
Toe off :		
FULL triple extension	Lacking hip and knee extension	1
Maximal arm drive backwards	Adequate	1
45–50° whole-body angle (first step), that rises with each step	Approx. 37°, would benefit from greater lean but body position ok	1
Head and neck leading forwards (horizontal, not dropping down)	Not perfect but not critical	1
Swing phase (rear portion):		
Active and rapid hip flexion recovery	Needs to be more purposeful	1
Horizontal shin with dorsi-flexed ankle	Good shin position, ankle neutral	2
Knee cross just after initial contact	Achieved	2
Swing phase (front portion):		
Active hip extension DOWNWARDS pre initial contact	Needs to be more down and less backward	1
Negative shin angle, placing the foot behind knee backwards into ground and under the stomach	Just about but more would be better	1
Total		14/24

separate successful professionals from the also-rans and nearly-made-its. Only once these phases have been completed can the player actually execute their move.

The CoD is inherently more varied than the acceleration and top-speed elements of running as it can be a subtle shift of momentum or a dramatic 180° turn. Despite this, there are still distinct phases of the task which must fulfil specific criteria in order to be effective. Each of these carries its own technical requirements, and is underpinned by different strength qualities.

Firstly there is a need to **decelerate**. Even a small change in direction will require a slight reduction in velocity. This is achieved through a shortening of the stride and a placing of the foot in front of the centre of mass (CoM). The more dramatic the change in direction, the greater the amount of deceleration required, and the further the foot needs to be placed outside of the CoM. By lowering the CoM the player is able to increase this distance more easily. This is often obvious during large cutting movements. However, even during more subtle shifts in direction a player will, entirely naturally, tend to lower their hips slightly.

Following the braking or deceleration step there comes the need to generate impulse in the desired direction of travel through the **active foot plant**. This foot contact also falls outside of the CoM in order to project horizontal force. In addition to correct positioning of the foot, this phase also requires a turning of the hips towards the new direction. The reason for this is two-fold. Firstly, it makes best mechanical use of the powerful hip extensors. Secondly it places the player in the correct position to execute the final phase. Extreme changes of direction can place significant demands on the ability to produce internal rotation of the hip. Consequently, poor performance of this skill or loss of form in the kinetic chain may often be the result of a lack of mobility in the hips.

Finally we have the **drive-off phase**. If the correct positions have been achieved in previous phases, then acceleration mechanics of straight-line running can be performed as the player starts to

What Does Agility Look Like?

When we think of agility training we tend to jump to images of poles and cones, generally laid out in a manner which demands repeated and dramatic shifts in direction from left to right. Aside from the previously mentioned lack of need to read stimuli or produce a rapid movement-response decision, this doesn't reflect the movements seen in the game.

Even the legendary mazy runs of Maradona featured small shifts of body weight to throw opponents off balance. I was once asked to collate some clips to illustrate what agility looked like in football. After a lot of trawling I came to the conclusion that by far the most common use of the skill comes from subtle shifts to throw an opponent off balance and create space to either run into or to execute a cross or shot.

This simply adds to the view that traditional SAQ-type agility training falls short when it comes to developing either the perceptual or mechanical skills set required to become more effective on the field of play.

re-accelerate in the new direction. While the previous deceleration should be kept to a minimum, that which is required should be performed as quickly as possible. The active foot plant will take the player from their slowest point into the new direction, and by turning the hips the player can now drive powerfully backwards and down to come out of the turn explosively.

10.7 Changing and Improving Running Technique

Any conversation around the adaptation of technique in running should begin with the acknowledgement that it is not a simple task. Even a young child has already 'rehearsed' many thousands of gait cycles while running, and so the motor pattern that we seek to change is highly engrained. Running 'technique' also occurs largely at a subconscious level, which makes it even harder to access. I place technique in inverted commas, as most people do not have a technique to speak of – they just run.

If we then consider an adult population with often low motivation and focus to improve technique, the task can start to seem impossible. Fear not, though: there are things we can do that are effective and reliable when used as part of a well-planned system.

One thing it is important to realise is that a large number of technical issues in running form arise from physical deficiencies, for example, a lack of local muscular conditioning to hold form for prolonged periods, restriction in certain structures causing misalignment or limited range of movement, etc. Therefore by addressing these we can get some quick wins (although this doesn't happen without good planning).

In terms of our coaching approach (think back to Chapter 3 and Systems of Delivery) we must remember the nature of the athlete we are working with. The majority of players are not highly motivated to work on technique, and coach:player ratios are generally insufficient for high-quality instruction to be given. Of course, it is possible to work individually outside of squad training sessions although this requires good, long-term commitment from the player. This also misses out on the opportunity to have a wide impact on the squad as a whole. Given that running technique is suboptimal in the vast majority of players and can aid both injury prevention, movement economy and enhance absolute performance, this seems too good an opportunity to let slip by.

When we think of making changing to running technique, the first approach is often to lift the coaching model straight from athletics. This often means a combination of running drills and rehearsed elements of sprinting with verbal feedback after each repetition. Of course, all the technical feedback in the world cannot help if a player doesn't have the physical capacity to produce these shapes. Furthermore, when given specific instructions the player is then required to make a conscious effort to adapt his technique in subsequent sprints. This is not particularly effective in the short term, as conscious movements must be somehow assimilated into subconscious patterns. In the longer term with regard to skill retention our results are likely to be poor as this conscious effort to change which is present during coached running is absent during games. I have had to learn the hard way through experience that it is possible over time to get a player moving really well during track sessions but then look like the two of you have never met during the match! If coaching cues are used they should certainly be extrinsic rather than intrinsic wherever possible. This means that the player should be instructed as to the outcome on the environment rather than the internal effort. An example would be, 'smash your foot into the floor', rather than 'drive down hard with your glutes'.

So in summary, 'unconscious learning' may be the most effective method of gaining running skill, and physical changes which underpin technique are as important as skill gains themselves. This leads us to a position whereby coaching by stealth or constraints-based coaching are ideally suited. Through intelligent exercise selection and well-planned constraints we can strengthen, mobilise and coordinate the patterns that will enable the player to run technically better. It is genuinely possible to have a running technique and speed-development programme without the players even being aware of it.

On the face of it this sounds incredibly easy. However, in order to be effective there are several things the S&C coach must know:

1. Which element of technique they want to target

2. What the current limiting factors to achieving this are (i.e. strength, mobility, skill, etc.)

3. Which drills or exercises are most effective at addressing these goals

The first of these phases is informed by a running assessment. Hopefully the process outlined earlier in this chapter which identifies the critical elements of technique and provides a framework for analysis, will aid the S&C coach in identifying the correct and most impactful elements of technique to address.

The second phase is the one which often distinguishes the novice from the expert. It is easy to stand on the touchline and play 'spot the error' in a player's running style. All too often simply telling the player what they need to do differently is wrongly passed off as coaching. Highly effective and insightful coaches are able to see a flaw and through past experience, knowledge of functional anatomy, and sometimes supplementary testing, identify the root cause behind it. There are many

possible explanations for a given technical issue, far beyond the scope of this book to evaluate in any detail. However, for a greater understanding I would direct you towards Bosch and Klomp's excellent book or the work of Ralph Mann.

Finally, once the issue and its causes have been diagnosed then an intervention can be selected. Ironically, this should in fact be a very simple task if the first two phases have been properly understood. There is no perfect recipe. Often a drill which one coach finds highly effective will be considered useless by another. Similarly some athletes will make huge gains with a drill that is totally ineffective with others. If the previous elements of the coaching process are a science, this is where the art comes to the fore. A degree of experimentation is required and the coach must have a clear vision of what they wish to achieve, and a good reflective process to ensure that their chosen method has been effective.

As another example of the value of working with good people, the best model which I have seen to describe the coaching thought process was sketched out over a lunch break by Jared Deacon – an excellent S&C and sprints coach. Jared's thought process (overleaf in Figure 10.7) clearly and simply illustrates the complex thought process and maturity of understanding context that goes into effective coaching.

The programme prescription, or coaching toolbox as it is described in the model on page 103, can be broken down into a number of subcategories:

- Isolated conditioning

- Isolated mobility

- Integrated conditioning

- Integrated mobility

- Intervention sprints

Isolated conditioning is appropriate when the raw ingredients are not sufficient. For example, a player may lack the basic trunk strength to hold form and resist lumbar extension when running at speed. Although technical work may help them to better utilise the strength they already possess, it may also be effective to strip things down and just develop the muscle. In this example an exercise such as Aleknas (see Chapter 7) would represent a good isolated exercise choice, as the target musculature is hit through a task which replicates

function. This is an important detail. The point of isolated work is to allow an overload of specific tissues to a greater extent than is possible in gross movements. However, where possible this reductionism should not be at the cost of function. So, to continue the example, an exercise choice such as sit-ups would work very similar tissues, but the task (dynamic trunk flexion) poorly represents the activity we are trying to improve. Therefore while the short-term goal of strengthening the trunk flexors may be achieved, our wider long-term goal is poorly served.

Isolated mobility work will often be required to address issues around posture. A lack of mobility

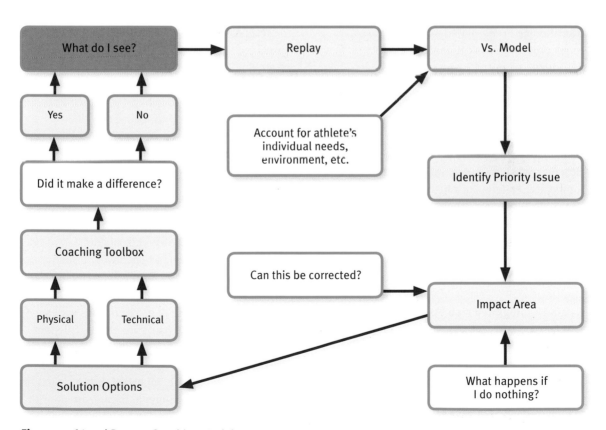

Figure 10.6 Jared Deacon Coaching Model

103

in the structures around the hips and thoracic spine are very common, and place non-negotiable limits on form. Great gains can be made in this area with a little dedication and commitment. Anyone who is interested in the area should head straight for Kelly Starrett's fantastic book, *Becoming a Supple Leopard*. This utilises a vast range of techniques to develop mobility and tissue quality.

Integrated conditioning involves highly specific movements, often elements of running themselves, with a focus on developing the physical capacity to perform a movement. Such tasks develop strength qualities, but also demand that they are matched by the skill to utilise them within the running cycle. Consequently they can also be effective when transitioning from isolated work or as part of a rehab process. Classic running drills, such as Mach ABC drills, can even be considered to fall into this category. While some may disagree, it is mine and many track coaches' view that to perceive these as skill practice is a misunderstanding. The skill transfer from these controlled, slower-paced drills to high-speed running is highly questionable. However, what is not debatable is that they allow for the accumulation of a higher volume of controllable practice of holding excellent form. Plyometrics may also be considered integrated conditioning, as the high skill and specificity of jumps and bounding work serve as an excellent bridge between the gym and pitch.

Similarly, **integrated mobility** moves away from purely structural limitations and introduces motor control through larger movement patterns. Here we are talking about training methods such as squat and lunge patterns and hurdle drills. The crucial component of effective practice here is to set the exercise up to ensure that mobility is achieved in the target area rather than through a compensation pattern. For example, squats can be effective in developing hip and ankle mobility – but only if the player's weight distribution is correct. If during the descent the weight is allowed to freely shift towards the front of the foot, then the tissues around the ankles will not be forced to adapt to a stress. Therefore, either effective cueing or creative use of constraints are required to make sure the outcome goal is achieved.

'Intervention sprints' is a term I would use to describe constraint-based running. Personally I feel that these are absolutely the key to making technical improvements in football players. Given that it is a form of coaching by stealth, it ticks all of the boxes in terms of ensuring that learning takes places on a subconscious, involuntary level. When constructed properly it ensures that the correct technical positions are achieved without exception. This means that it is suddenly possible to work with a large group of players with poor attention focus and still achieve your technical outcome consistently throughout the group. Finally, conditioning and mobilisation occurs through appropriate patterns, as the opportunity to compensate has been removed.

10.8 Practical Drills

I firmly believe that the essence of good technical coaching comes from having a sound understanding of exactly what you are trying to change, and the mechanism by which you will achieve it. The practice of great coaches varies enormously, but these traits are always constant. So far I have attempted to provide a framework for understanding what good technique looks like, why these positions are important, and a structure of working to effect change. In theory, armed with those tools the task of designing interventions should be relatively simple. All that said, it is

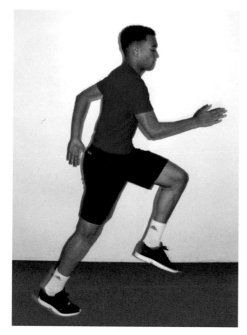

Drill-to-Sprint Combination

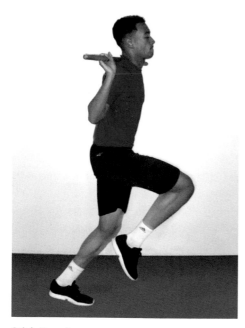

Stick Running

footballers is stick running. As the name suggests, this involves running with a stick across the shoulders, as in a back squat. When a player is in full hip extension at toe off, any further movement of the leg to the rear cannot come from extension but instead from rotation of the pelvis. The essence of this drill is that given the limited capacity for rotation, or rather return from rotation, the player is forced to bring the thigh through hip flexion earlier.

If you have read this chapter so far you will immediately recognise that this will promote front-side mechanics, and will also know why this is desirable. The capacity of this simple drill to reduce pendulum swing and place the player in a position to apply downward thrust is quite remarkable. Almost without exception I have found this simple intervention to improve mechanics immediately without any verbal instruction. What's more, players typically report back that they feel quicker and are all of a sudden exposed to a new feeling of movement, which can start to re-programme their instinct. Fans of dynamical systems theory would describe this as developing a new attractor state. The only caveat is that they must be running with sufficient intensity that they have to adapt to the drill and must try to keep facing forwards.

No-Arms Running

No-arms running is essentially the same drill as stick running. In an ideal world I would slightly favour stick running, as the length of the stick has a greater capacity to limit rotation. However, no-arms running can be more practical with larger groups as no equipment is required.

Step-Over Drills

These are a fantastic tool for promoting a really positive first step in acceleration, during which

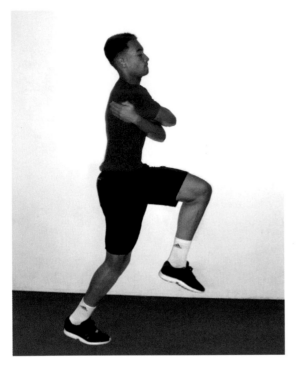

No-Arms Running

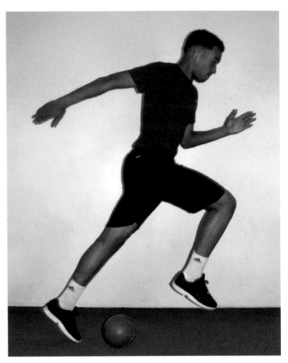

Step-Over Drills

the player exerts a powerful downward and backward thrust. What is interesting is that only a handful of these obstacles need to be used in order to affect the rest of the run. It seems that once the positive pattern is set, players generally continue to run in this way for the rest of the given sprint. Indeed, it is even possible to use a single obstacle to change the initial step and still see results thereafter. Once again, when working in large groups of varied stride length, this can be quite important. On a practical level, it is possible to use a ball as a cue for the first step, as in the illustration below. I would concede that these drills may be considered contrary to the technical model of keeping the foot low to the ground during acceleration. However, the goal is not to replicate the technique perfectly, but rather to

promote a hip- and quad-dominant downward thrust in the classic 'piston action', rather than a hamstring-dominant pulling action which is often seen.

Sled Running

Sled running is generally regarded as a way to add resistance to the sprinting action and is therefore a highly specific form of weight training. However, it can also be used to help players to experience the correct body position during acceleration. It is a common technical error for players to achieve a 'false angle' whereby they flex at the hip. This means that rather than producing the 45–50° lean through the whole body, they place themselves in a position which prevents a full triple extension. The weight of the sled makes it much easier to find

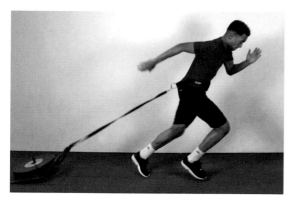

Sled Running

this position without fear of losing balance. This is not the whole picture, as without the sled the player still requires sufficient stiffness at the knee to hold form. The sled still provides a good alternative to trying to describe the lean through verbal cueing, which can often produce some hideous results.

Another technical benefit to the sled is it promotes a longer, more forceful ground contact. This is often overlooked. At top speed the goal is to achieve brief ground contacts to avoid braking, and take advantage of opportunity for elastic energy. However, this is reversed during acceleration. As the player has little or no velocity, the danger of braking impulse is far lower. Similarly, the potential for elastic energy is lower and concentric power production becomes much more significant (see Chapter 11). Therefore the technique adopted must be geared towards creating as much impulse as possible. This means high forces for as long as possible. It is a classic mistake to confuse cadence with speed during acceleration. The tell-tale sign of this comes when a player appears to be moving their feet very quickly but going nowhere.

Sprints with no Interventions

All of the above represent drills whereby different types of intervention sprints have been used to help players gain greater technical proficiency through conditioning, to support good technique and enforced exposure to correct pattering. On that basis it would be remiss not to mention good old-fashioned sprints themselves. A funny thing happens when we sprint – we naturally start to run better. All of a sudden knee lift starts to increase. Stiffness around the knee increases and ground contact times shorten. The trunk becomes more stable and resists rotation. Because so many technical errors come from the fact that a player does not have the strength to work correctly, running hard can provide them with that strength. I believe there is also an element of subconscious self-coaching. Good athletes find ways to move effectively and efficiently. If they are exposed to good volumes of sprinting, they will naturally start to self-optimise and find more effective ways of moving through natural adaptation.

011
improving speed
in the weight room

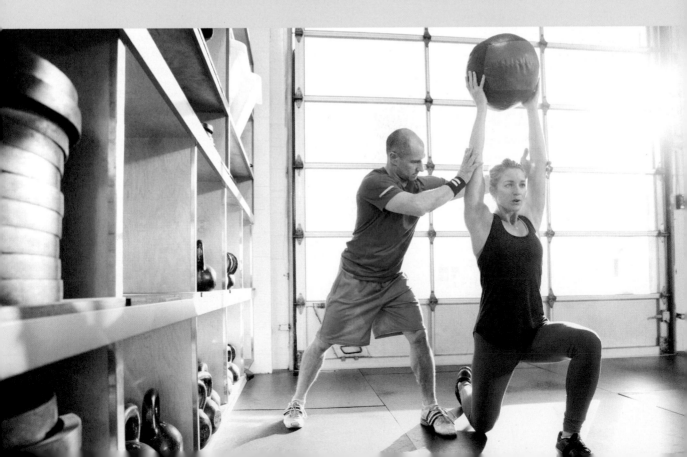

For all the many ways in which speed can be enhanced by changing mechanics, it is often the case that giving a player a bigger engine is the quickest and most effective way of making speed gains. This standpoint comes from the fact that the rapid expression of force is one of the most important indicators of a player's ability to move effectively. As legendary sprints coach Charlie Francis puts it, '*To go faster you need more force*', or Lauren Seagrave, '*The key to speed is applying large forces over short periods of time.*'

If we are comfortable with the efficacy of changes to running mechanics being supported by a belief that players generally do not move very well, a similar situation exists with increasing force production capacity. Almost without exception, football players are not strong. Now, before I am assaulted with examples of players with great strength, I must frame that comment. Of course many players exhibit natural strength and at levels beyond the general population or their colleagues, but this does not make them truly strong. The nature of training programmes and the culture of the sport dictate that the gap between a player's genetic ceiling for strength and their actual levels is always considerable. On that basis alone, there is always likely to be opportunity for gains in strength and speed through well-planned strength training.

Hopefully it is not necessary to point out to the reader of this book that force can be expressed and measured in many ways. This may refer to the type of muscle contraction (eccentric, isometric, concentric), relative versus absolute force, rate of force development versus maximum force, kinematics, etc. Consequently we need to match strength-training methods to the nature of force production in the action we are seeking to enhance (i.e. acceleration, CoD, etc.).

If we begin with the initiation of a sprint, **acceleration** is chiefly determined by relative concentric peak force expressed over the brief ground contact time available. The most natural assessment of this would come in the form of jump testing. Traditional resistance-training methods are limited by concentric force production (i.e. can you lift the bar back up, rather than can you lower it). Therefore, when combined with loaded explosive work and jump training, these tools are well-suited to developing the qualities which underpin acceleration. It should be noted that this analysis relates to a pure acceleration, that is to say, one which starts from zero velocity. This may be from a standing start or following a dramatic change in direction whereby speed has dropped close to or to zero. However, many accelerations in football occur from jogging or running, and therefore the qualities become a blend of pure acceleration and maximum speed.

The nature of force production during **maximum speed running** is very different to acceleration. In this instance, rather than generating large concentric forces to produce velocity, the challenge is the reuse of energy. Therefore it is not surprising that stretch-shortening cycle, or reactive strength and maximum absolute strength appear most related to maximum speed. It is also important to understand that these two qualities act in tandem, as maximum strength is important to maintain stiffness about the knee to avoid yielding and take advantage of the potential for elastic recoil. The nature of these force qualities mean that while gym-based resistance training is still important, it is probably best considered a building block towards more specific work with a greater bias on reactive strength, such as sprints and plyometrics.

When it comes to **changes of direction** and strength training, the picture has remained unclear for many years. Unlike straight-line running, CoD involves many distinct phases each with their own characteristics. Furthermore, the successful performance of these tasks is greatly influenced by cognitive skills, such as the reading of visual cues and the experience to select the correct movement response. As a result, researchers have found it a challenge to relate strength qualities to agility. The multi-factorial nature of the challenge is reflected in the fact that reactive strength, maximal dynamic, isometric, concentric and eccentric strength have all been shown to be related. However, recent studies have suggested that, while many are related, eccentric strength is the sole predictor of change of direction performance. Of course, the effectiveness of the mechanics used by the player will affect their ability to produce force, and vice-versa. Players with greater relative lower-body strength produce greater foot-plant forces and faster change of direction performances, but this is in part achieved by having the strength to maintain optimal mechanics.

Agility – The Importance of Flow

As we've seen, the production and control of force is clearly vital for effective changes of direction and general agility. However, there is a paradoxical view whereby the most effective player is not the one who can produce the most force, but the one who can produce the same movement with the LEAST force. As you will go on to read in Chapter 12, there are players who possess great straight-line speed and force capacity, but who always disappoint when it comes to changing direction. Typically, these players lack what I call 'flow'. That relaxed, balanced strength and coordination, that ability to use the postural muscles rather than prime movers, is what these players lack.

This is worth bearing in mind if weight room training of strength does not seem to be impacting on agility. Flow is certainly a trainable quality. However, this may be a case of, 'not everything which can be measured counts, and not everything which counts can be measured'.

11.1 Developing Strength Qualities for Speed

The research discussed above gives a clear guide as to the specific strength qualities which underpin speed and agility. However, being overly specific too early and too often is an easy but dangerous trap to fall into.

General Preparatory Work

Although it is not well-represented in the scientific literature, any coach worth their salt knows that a good movement base is the requisite platform for building strength qualities. Over the years I have come to learn that resistance training is most effective when used first as a tool for improving quality of movement, and then improving quantity. I can back this up with countless examples of Olympic athletes and professional footballers who have improved performance without adding a single kilo to the bar. It makes sense that a player should unlock and fully utilise their existing strength before adding more capacity to an inefficient system. This could be viewed as using lifting as a motor control and mobility programme first, and a strength-training modality second.

In reality this can simply mean doing the basics very well. This can be a tricky concept to sell, as it is something which almost every coach in the world thinks they already do (which is patently not the case). Simple movement patterns based primarily around bilateral and unilateral squat patterns (including dead lifts), combined with good jump skills, are an essential foundation before we begin to load the bar. The latter of these in particular is often overlooked. It still baffles me that so many coaches go to great lengths to become as expert as possible in coaching Olympic lifts, but remain novice at such a fundamental expression of relative force as jumping.

Bilateral squat patterns must be developed through full range and with excellent control. This is particularly important when we consider that a longer muscle fibre can contract at a greater velocity than a shorter fibre (due to sarcomeres in series). It has recently been demonstrated that the enhancement of force production and jump performance is as effective, if not more so, with deep versus half-squatting. This therefore ends any sensible debate that only partial-range squatting is required. Unilateral patterns need to be performed with unwavering stability, an appropriate trunk position to take advantage of the power of the hips and with excellent control of trunk stability in all planes. Jump skills need to be performed with an appropriate kinetic-chain sequence (i.e. hip, knee, toe), with good stability, appropriate foot contact position and joint angles matched to the task (i.e. shallow knee and hip angle during brief ground contacts and increasing angle with duration).

Unfortunately it is common to see squat patterns assessed through a handful of unloaded repetitions free from fatigue, and a jump judged solely on the basis of flight time. A more robust measure of movement requires assessment of patterns with moderate loading, performed repeatedly, sometimes with fatigue. We need to know more than just what the player can do as a one-off under easy conditions. The jump needs to be assessed not just from the outcome (i.e. height jumped), but also in terms of how it was produced.

To improve these patterns we require *some* load. If we simply perform the movements free from loading there is insufficient stimulus for the tissues and the nervous system to adapt (i.e. overload – one of the first principles of S&C). Here's the big problem though: the load required is only relatively moderate. This may not seem an issue, most sensible coaches start off with moderate loading. However, what you do or don't do next is an absolutely critical stage in the process. The average coach keeps this player in a safe but not perfect window of technique. Because they have not clearly determined their thought process regarding performance enhancement, the next step is to start to increase the load. This they do. The technique remains safe but may break down a little, and range-of-movement may decrease a little ... and now we're in trouble. The opportunity to enhance movement quality has been lost, as we have compromised technique, albeit to a subtle degree. This has been done in the belief that more weight will mean more strength, and thus force, and thus speed.

In my experience, loads of as little as around 40–50kg during bilateral lifts and 20–30kg during unilateral lifts are sufficient to provide stimulus for movement enhancement. Of course, more can be better – but only if the quality of movement is maintained. The problem comes from the belief that moving outside of this range means strength gains.

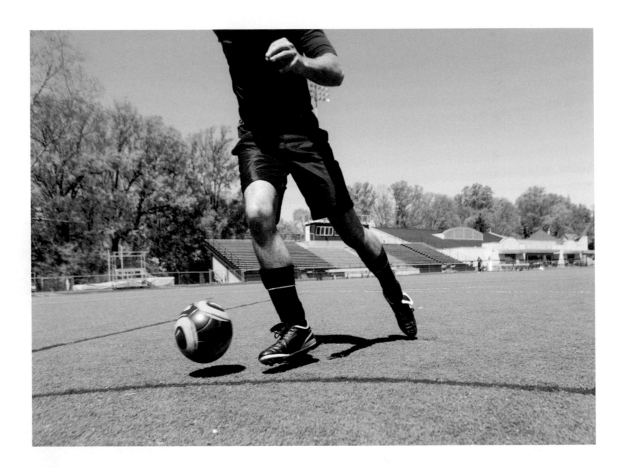

A player running at these speeds is able to produce massive amounts of force very rapidly. Do we really think that an 80kg squat will overload the force production capacity of a player who can run in excess of 30km/h? Don't get me wrong, I'm all for adding load, and an 80kg squat through full ROM with good control is something I would encourage. But an 80kg squat with compromised control and partial range is what I think of as the 'dead zone' of football S&C. The player has moved away from developing their movement quality and is not stimulated enough to enhance the engine size. Instead they have fallen into the trap of just doing 'stuff'. They will feel like they have worked hard. They may have some DOMS in their legs,

they will feel a little fatigued and will be pleased to have added load. Sadly though, the precise approach to truly understanding targeted adaptation and performance impact has been lost. The load will likely plateau relatively soon due to the demands of training, and the quality will remain static.

Let's take a more optimistic view. What happens if we rewind the clock to the crossroads where the coach added load. If, instead of adding load, the depth was increased a little, or cues were added to make the movement even more solid, then maybe we have taken an opportunity to do something different. I've been lucky to work with one of the best strength coaches going for many years, Arun Singh. I have also observed lots of very average S&C coaches. Despite having trained people to incredible levels of strength (including a world record 400+kg squat) Arun would always spend far longer keeping athletes on lighter loads than the average coaches. He understood that you only get one chance to develop a base of excellence in movement. If you play your hand too soon, it's gone. Think of it as the tortoise and the hare. Consider the weights lifted by most of the players you work with. How long does it take to achieve those loads? Weeks maybe, months at most. The moral of the story is, perfectionism and low load beats high load and compromise.

Specific Preparatory Work

The consideration of specific strength qualities comes having 'unlocked' the athletic potential of a player and provided a solid basis for genuine strength training through development of range and control in fundamental patterns.

We face an interesting dilemma with regard to how much emphasis we place on strength versus power training. To a great extent this is very much a matter of personal philosophy and what works within your own system. I think it is too extreme to suggest that there is a right or a wrong way. However, the work of Prue Cormie in recent years has provided some useful insight into how strength-trained athletes differ in their responses when compared with weaker ones. This work can be explained simplistically in that strength training provides us with more force-production material, whereas power training optimises our strategy for utilising this material. Strong athletes appear to respond better to power training than weaker athletes. Essentially this is because there is greater opportunity to optimise a large-force production capacity. If you have little strength,

using it more efficiently will have limited effectiveness.

Another argument for initially favouring strength over power is that by seeking a general upshift in the force–velocity curve, all of the distinct elements of strength which we have discussed with regard to running and CoD will be positively affected. Some may argue that just getting strong will not directly transfer to speed, and even cite literature studies to prove the point. Their argument is supported by the fact that slow, bilateral strength exercises are so dramatically different in terms of motor pattern and kinematics that the idea of transfer to sprinting is naïve. And they would probably be right … if it weren't for the fact that no player just does strength training in isolation. When they next go out on to the training pitch they perform a large volume of specific strength work in the form of sprinting, cutting and jumping. The analogy I like to use to explain my philosophy is that of the dinner party. The work we do in the gym is like the trip to the supermarket. Here we are just acquiring our ingredients. This is important as we need more raw material but we cannot possibly just serve this up and call it a dinner party. The training pitch is the kitchen. It is through all the highly specific, 'disguised strength training' while on the training pitch that the work we did in the gym starts to pay dividends. Finally, the match itself is the dinner party where we can produce the finished article of speed and power in its completed form. It should be noted that recent studies suggest that the direct transfer of strength gains to speed is much more effective in those with low-strength training backgrounds (i.e. most footballers).

I do not want to appear overly dogmatic though, or suggest that strength and power boils down to an either/or argument. To my mind both should be present within the training programme at pretty much all times. It simply comes down to where the biggest emphasis lies. I personally find that the use of jumps and sprints within complexes helps to aid the transfer of strength training, and reduces the shift in motor pattern which the player has to face in the subsequent pitch session. In reality, a flowing back and forth between the two biases is probably best practice. Variety of stimulus is far more important than performing a perceived optimal blend constantly.

We have already discussed the specific strength qualities which underpin the various components of sprint running in football. These are summarised and matched to appropriate training methods in Table 11.1 below.

It may seem that the natural progression in our discussion here is to begin to unpack these broad headlines I have used to describe training methods and get into the level of exercise details. However,

for me, that is an inappropriate. The essence of good S&C is the ability to be highly individualised and targeted. I may have three players in the gym, who play for the same team and have the same goal of improving peak force to help their acceleration. Does this mean they all do the same programme? Absolutely not. Even when their programmes look the same, they probably won't be, but the devil is in the detail. I could have all of these players performing squats for 5 sets of 5 reps. However, subtle differences may mean that they utilise different types of squat, receive different cues, etc. Hopefully this illustrates why it would be foolish to start to try to get to this level of prescription within a book.

For years, S&C coaches have debated about methods of training and particularly exercise selection. The use of bilateral squats versus unilateral. Do you coach Olympic lifts to footballers or opt for the less-technical jump squats? I hope I can end this debate with the following simple statements:

Table 11.1	Strength Qualities Underpinning Sprint Running & CoD and Associated Training Methods	
Action	**Underpinning Qualities**	**Suitable Methods**
Acceleration	Relative concentric peak force	• Traditional strength training to enhance peak force • Ballistic jump work to develop concentric power • Explosive power training
Maximum Speed	Reactive strength, maximum absolute strength	• Sprints and plyometrics for stiffness and reactive strength • Maximum strength training for absolute force production
Change of direction	Eccentric strength and reactive strength	• Plyometrics for reactive strength and eccentric strength (with a specific focus on accepting landing for eccentric strength)

- If you want them to develop strength … find a movement that allows the player to express force maximally and train it.

- If you want them to develop power … find a movement that allows them to express force explosively and train it.

Anyone who feels we need to be more prescriptive than that has missed the point. My personal preference is not to use Olympic lifts in football, certainly not on a wholesale basis. This is based purely on the time burden and the difficulty in being effective in coaching them. That is certainly not to say it can't be done. If a coach values it highly enough, has a coaching method which produces good technique and understands the adaptations they achieve and how they fit into a philosophy, then power to them.

Plyometrics is a subject which is close to my heart as it has been the subject of my PhD. The application of plyometrics in football poses a lot of questions. I think a good starting point comes from the following passage in Verkoshanky and Siff's *Supertraining*:

> *More often than not, plyometric enthusiasts do not consider the possibility that the athlete's sport alone may offer all or most of the plyometric training that is necessary and that adding more of this type of loading may be excessive or unwarranted.*

This reflects what we have already discussed in terms of 'on-pitch strength training'. The key is that rather than just assuming this has taken place, we ideally need to be able to measure and control the number of jumps, sprints, turns, etc., which a player performs. In the event that we do decide that an additional plyometric stimulus is

Transmission vs. Generation

Discussions around production of force tend to lead to thought processes and training methods which centre around the generation of force at the joint. However, what actually counts when it comes to performance is the application of this force into the ground. The key to linking these and ensuring the former impacts on the latter is the effective transmission of force.

Stiffness in the ankles and knees is an absolute fundamental of effective sprint running. Try watching the slow motion replay of a 100m race and see how little give occurs at the ankles, despite huge forces being transmitted through them. Strength training can certainly help to develop some of the ingredients of stability and even have a direct impact itself. However, sprint running and plyometric activities are the best natural fit for making sure that what starts at the joints sees its way all the way through to the ground without leaking.

required, the choice of exercise can be an interesting area. In the past I have conducted research which suggested that classic plyometrics did not offer any advantage in terms of intensity over activities performed as part of sports performance. To test this theory, I looked at what happens when a player performs typical single-leg plyometric exercises such as vertical and horizontal hopping, in comparison with leaping to head a ball. Players performed each of these with ground-reaction forces measured via a force plate. The results are illustrated in Figure 11.1, page 116. This shows quite nicely how closely matched all three tasks were in terms of the propulsive forces involved, the length of ground contact and the total force applied (impulse). The initial spike at the beginning of both of the plyometric exercises is the impact force on initial contact. It could be argued that this is useful for increasing the total mechanical load on a player and developing their capacity to resist yielding. What is clear though is that the use of more specific tasks, such as leaping to head a ball, allow the player to express propulsive force just as well as traditional exercises. The advantage of these is that player motivation and engagement are likely to be higher, and the transfer of skill is also likely to be greater.

So, having come up with a clear philosophy around exercise selection, we can now get down to the nuts and bolts and programming – set and rep protocols. We could cover the well-trodden ground of describing the typical ranges used for strength versus power versus hypertrophy, etc. That seems somewhat pointless though, as it has been covered countless times in other textbooks.

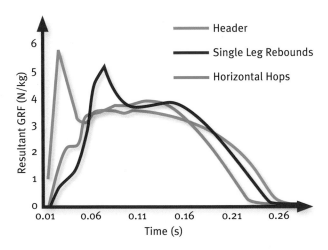

Figure 11.2 Traditional Plyometrics vs. Typical Game Activity
Source: Jarvis pilot data (unpublished)

More to the point though, it may also take us away from the fundamental view of individualisation. A landmark study a few years ago illustrated clearly how the adaptations to different protocols, both in terms of hormonal response and performance changes, were highly individual. This shatters the concept that a player may begin training in higher rep ranges, say 4 sets of 10 at 70% 1 rep max, but will have to progress to lower volumes and higher loads, such as 5 sets of 5 at 85% in order to get stronger. Of course, this is not an all-or-nothing debate. Once again, variety of stimulus may be more important than the perfect set–rep configuration. The important message is that we need to evaluate and monitor what is working for an individual player and programme accordingly, rather than looking to a menu to programme for us.

Special Preparatory Work

The natural choices for special preparatory exercises with regard to sprinting are sprinting itself and resisted sprinting. It seems fitting that these are the last two modalities which we discussed with regard to making technical changes. This fits perfectly with the concept that special preparatory work combines strength qualities with technical skill, and squares the circle on our training philosophy.

Resisted sprinting, such as with a sled or a bungee cord, can be a good tool for developing strength qualities in a closely matched motor pattern as well as teaching a player to express force effectively. Often this is limited in free sprinting due to a desire to achieve a high cadence to the cost of force production. Concerns that the change in the motor pattern may have negative consequences are allayed by the findings that sled and free sprinting combined can produce superior gains than free sprinting alone.

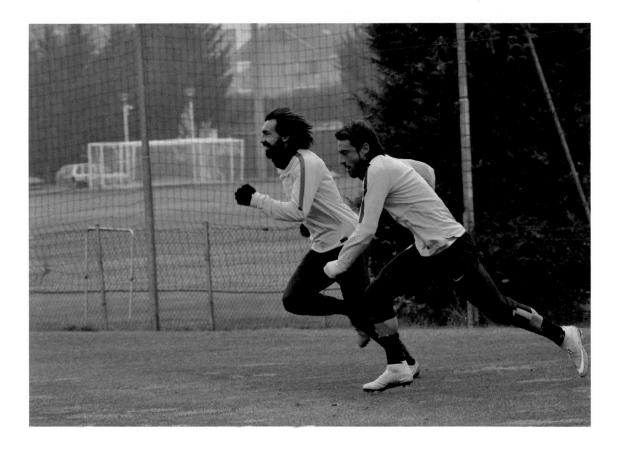

I once heard someone at an S&C conference ask a speaker what the best exercise for football is. This is clearly a ridiculous question. However, if I had to answer it I might well come back with sprinting as a reasonable response. If you want to make a player quicker, make them practise running quickly. It doesn't need to be the only thing you do, but it will certainly give you the biggest bang for your buck. The other thing worth bearing in mind is to make them run against quick people. Every decent sprints coach in the world knows that if you want to run really fast, you have to train with fast people. There's no getting around it. For your slower players this won't be a problem. However, for the quickest players, the chances are they will not maximise their gains from sprint work unless you handicap the distances or start times to make sure they have to go all out. Effort is everything.

11.2 Summary

Once injury reduction and player availability has been addressed, the biggest opportunity to enhance performance for an S&C coach lies in affecting how a player moves about the pitch. This may come in the form of greater efficiency for energy conservation and reduction of mechanical stress, or in terms of maximising speed and agility. The challenge is certainly not a simple one, but with an analytical mindset and a clear philosophy there is a huge opportunity to add to a player's performance and the potential success of the team.

012
upper-body and
trunk training

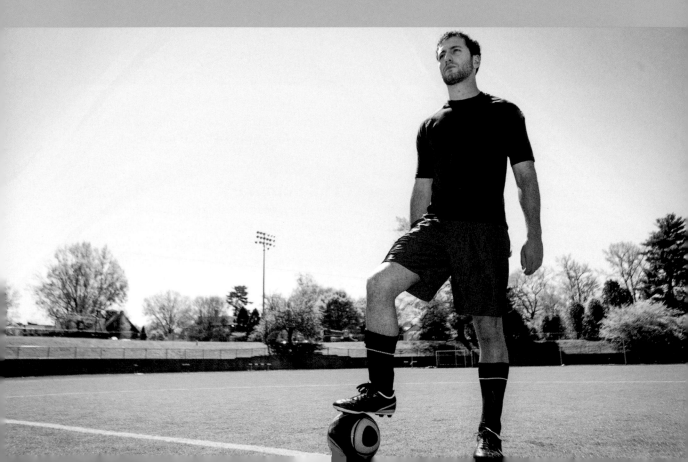

The case for true upper-body training to enhance performance is pretty flimsy. It is sometimes utilised as a tool for players who need to get better at holding off an opponent. However, a simple analysis of the movement makes it clear that it is not the arms and shoulders which limit this ability but the trunk, balance and the ability to set-up a stable base of support. On other occasions the need for upper-body strength may be attributed to the need for greater height when leaping. I have spent a great deal of time working with Olympic-level high jumpers, and a quick look at their physique confirms that they never touch a bench press. We have also discussed in earlier chapters that the role of the arms in running velocity is highly overstated.

So, does that mean the argument is finally put to bed? All bench presses, dumbbells and pull-up bars can be sold off and never seen again in football? Not quite. There is a need to be a bit more pragmatic here for a number of reasons. For one thing, a lot of upper-body exercises are excellent for training the trunk and therefore CAN help to develop the ability to hold off an opponent (such as press-ups). The difference here is that while the arms are responsible for the movement it is the trunk that is the target of our intentions. Therefore the term 'upper-body training' is somewhat deceptive. We should also consider that the body is not made up of isolated body parts with no interaction. Weakness or tightness in one area can have implications far away in the body. If a player has poor thoracic posture (i.e. kyphosis), this may lead to dysfunction further down the posterior chain and increase his risk of problems such as hamstring injury. Upper-body training has the potential to correct such issues, and therefore can contribute to enhanced global movement. Of course, it should also be noted that inappropriate upper-body training can also do the reverse, such as create or increase kyphosis and internally

rotated humerus, from an anterior-dominated programme (aka mirror training).

In reality, a great deal of the upper-body training which goes on in football club gyms throughout the land has got absolutely nothing to do with performance. So-called 'beach weights', i.e. exercise intended to make you look good on the beach, are pretty much ubiquitous. This has frustrated no end of S&C coaches who look across the gym wanting to see a performance environment but instead find what looks like a bodybuilding club. The thing is, though, boys will be boys – and that's not necessarily a bad thing. (Incidentally, girls will be girls too and the desire for 'guns' is not gender-specific if you think I'm discriminating.) We have all experienced the feeling of walking out of the gym with our body image suitably heightened. To everyone else we look exactly the same but we FEEL different. Players are the same. It may be that if we step back and think of them on a human level, there may actually be a performance gain to be found after all.

I can think of one player in particular who was very slightly smaller than average. This didn't ever seem to affect his game, but it definitely affected his psyche. His self-image seemed to be of a much smaller man, and that affected him negatively. If he stood in the tunnel and saw a bigger player, his confidence would drop. Now, while a bench-press session and some mirror posing clearly had no positive effective on any of our traditional markers of performance, I believe they could be very potent for him. It is often said by psychologists that it is not what we see, but the eyes from which we see it that counts. In this example the opponent who had previously seemed dominating now seems less so. There are actually some well-established physiological phenomena which may occur in this type of situation to enhance performance. By boosting the confidence and self-image of the player, we have the opportunity to achieve a hormonal priming effect. This can play an important role in performance in physiological terms, such as improved force and power output, but also decision making and cognitive function. Along the same lines, as much as it doesn't always sit comfortably, the hyper-macho atmosphere of the 'bench-press club' may actually augment testosterone as well. As a result, what you lose in one element of training may boost another if your genuine performance-lifting or on-pitch work is carried out in a superior hormonal environment. This is a great example of how it can sometimes be wise to step away from our discipline and look at the bigger picture.

If then we can accept that some upper-body training may be permissible even if the specific muscular adaptations do not directly map to performance it seems a sensible strategy to at least guide players towards exercises which are likely to have the greatest degree of transfer. Typically this means multi-joint exercises with the trunk unsupported. This would include work such as press-ups, pull-ups, suspension trainer work and med ball drills. Olympic lifts can also potentially be considered in this category. During programming these choices can quickly start to seem repetitive if a creative approach is not taken. Therefore given that exercise selection may be somewhat limited, small variations in technique and creative manipulation of set/rep protocols and additional loading must be utilised.

The example of 'Positive Pollution' I described in Chapter 3 proved to be a highly effective method of shifting upper-body training culture. This involved arranging for a wall of suspension trainers to be permanently installed across one wall of the gym, while at the same time removing all bench-press options. I knew that left to their own devices the players would try a handful of

pressing and pulling movements before getting bored (the difficulty of not having weight to add as easily as a barbell). Therefore I took the very deliberate step of showing a couple of key players some tough exercise challenges. These included a handstand press-up and a wall press-up (feet into the wall and off the ground). These were tricky challenges at first, but achievable with a bit of practice. I then stood back and was happy to see exactly what I had hoped would happen occur. Once these influential players mastered the skill it looked quite impressive – prompting the naturally competitive colleagues to want to try too. Now all of a sudden nobody was complaining about a lack of bench press, but good numbers were coming in to work on their own and try to nail the skills. In one fell swoop the suitability of the exercise had been improved to target performance, and competition and challenge had remained.

Suspension Training

Suspension training and gymnastic-type work are obvious choices if we wish to target the trunk via upper-limb movements. As has already been suggested, a slightly different approach to training may be required when using this type of work. Although body weight can be offset through bands, and load can be added through vests, etc., the S&C coach still doesn't have the precision of load manipulation available during traditional weight training. This should not be considered a major limitation – it simply means that greater attention needs to be paid to other variables such as volume, recovery and speed of movement. Perhaps most importantly though, subtle shifts in mechanics can be used to affect the intensity rather than using load as the primary method of doing so. As an aside, this can actually be quite a healthy developmental exercise for an S&C coach to become more skilled at playing with these variables rather than relying on the number stamped on the plates. We all know people who go to the gym and have their favourite routine of press-ups and abdominal exercises. These people tend to work hard but never make any year-on-year progress. This is a trap which we can fall into with suspension training if close attention is not paid.

Imagination is the only limit to the number of ways in which an S&C coach can give a player their desired upper-body session while also developing global strength and athleticism. The examples below illustrate the type of options which I have found useful, and are merely suggestions as a starting point.

Table 12.1	Example Suspension Trainer Pressing Exercises

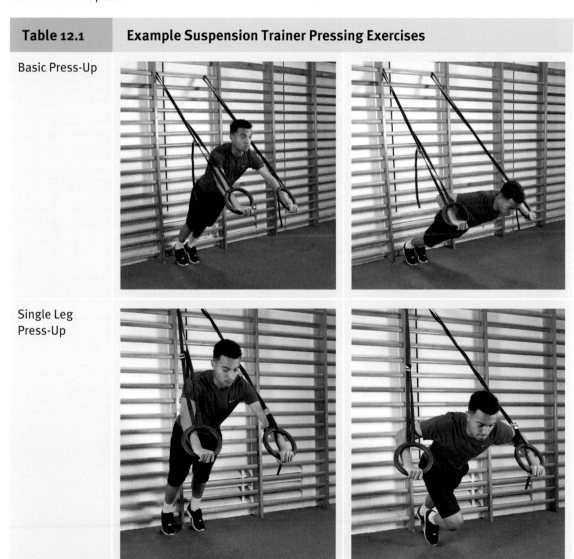

Basic Press-Up

Single Leg Press-Up

Table 12.1	Example Suspension Trainer Pressing Exercises (cont.)
Feet Suspended Press-Ups	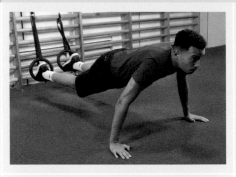 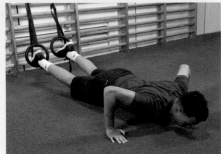
Weighted Press Up	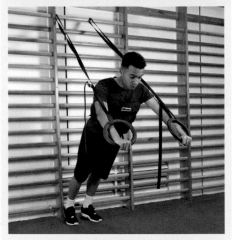 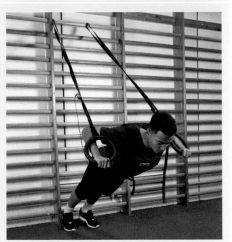
Single Arm Press Up	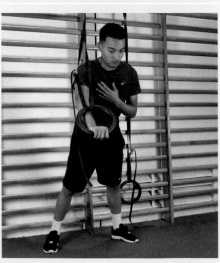 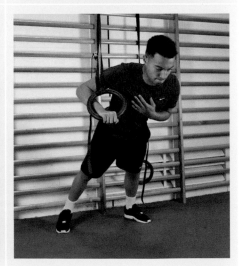

Table 12.1	Example Suspension Trainer Pressing Exercises (cont.)
Full Body Press Up	
Handstand Press Up	
Press Ups with hip flexion	

Table 12.1	Example Suspension Trainer Pressing Exercises (cont.)
Single Arm Press & Fly	
Crucifix Flys	
Crucifix Plank	

Table 12.2	Example Suspension Trainer Pulling Exercises

Reverse Flys

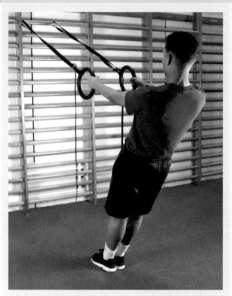 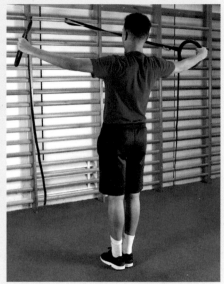

Inverse Pulls

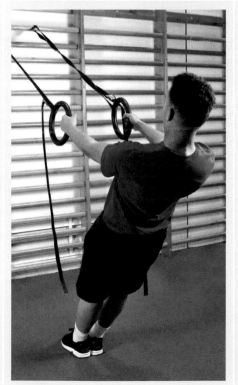 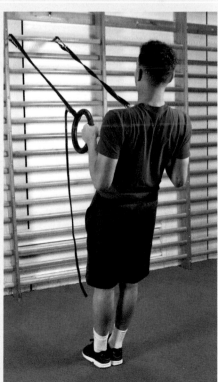

Table 12.2	Example Suspension Trainer Pulling Exercises (cont.)
Single Arm Inverse Pull	
Reverse Pull Up	

12.1 Trunk Training

In football, as in practically all sports, the trunk performs a pivotal role in all skills and locomotion. The trunk should provide effective transmission of forces from the limbs across the body in a manner which is both efficient and fluid. Poor trunk control will lead to a compromise in skills performance, will make movements less efficient/slower and will increase the risk of some of the most prevalent injuries such as hamstring and groin injuries, as a result of a lack of pelvic control.

It is important that the 'trunk' does not just mean the anterior abdominal musculature, but all aspects of the lower torso. It is also important to distinguish this term from the 'core' which includes components of the hip, groin, etc. Despite this it should also be remembered that many of these areas will have implications for trunk control. For example, poor thoracic mobility will inevitably compromise trunk stability when a player is attempting to move through full ROM.

Optimal trunk control requires both the basic muscular capacity to tolerate a load, as well as the specific neuromuscular skill to perform a task. Some players are able to develop high levels of skill and can therefore perform complex tasks with relative ease and without the need for high levels of local muscular strength. Similarly, players who move with efficient mechanics on the pitch will significantly reduce the forces which the trunk must tolerate. Conversely, there are players who exhibit high levels of muscular trunk strength in gym tasks, but fail to utilise this in play due to inefficient motor skills and/or poor movement patterns.

It is vital that the S&C programme recognises the different role of trunk musculature in training. The 'superficial abs' are naturally suited to producing/ tolerating high levels of force. This is vital for high-power actions such as sprinting, turning, etc. However, the deep abdominal musculature's function is to ensure low-level stability, control and posture. An overreliance on the superficial musculature will result in inefficient movement and excessive tension. Players commonly fail to utilise lower-level musculature effectively, and subsequently demonstrate poor movement and high risk of injury due to compromised lumbar–pelvic control. These players require low-level isolation exercises and motor control training. For this reason it is crucial that trunk training is not viewed as a continuum, with low levels being ignored once a player has 'graduated' from them. This type of scenario is illustrated in the example below:

'Dean' was a naturally strong, explosive and fast player with good athletic ability. He had good straight-line speed, but his CoD was considered poor. He had highly toned abdominals and was able to perform high-force tasks with relative comfort. Despite this he would consistently suffer from back spasms during 4-min steady runs in pre-season. During lower-level trunk tasks such as dead bugs he also found them tougher than expected and appeared to have dysfunctional patterns providing his stability (i.e. felt the work in his back, rather than his lower abdominals).

There was a Eureka moment when some of the other players described a session when they were stick wrestling and Dean was particularly poor. This was notable due to his significant upper-body musculature and obvious strength. It suggested to me that his inability to turn was most likely due to a heavy

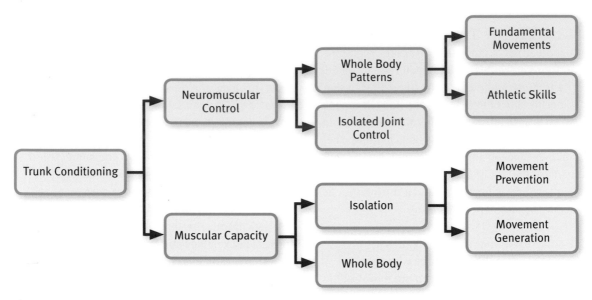

Figure 12.1 Trunk-Conditioning Model

reliance on superficial musculature, which resulted in him having to work excessively hard and ineffectively.

This is not to detract from the need for basic isolated strength. If the player does not have the raw capacity, then no level of skill will help them to control the trunk.

A conceptual model of trunk training is summarised in Figure 12.1, above.

12.2 Spinal Flexion Training and Safe Movements

In terms of maintaining spinal health, one of the key theories which has emerged in recent years is that of sparing spinal flexions. This is based on the theory that micro-damage occurs to the intervertebral discs during flexion, and that each athlete's spine has a finite number of flexions before injury occurs. On this basis, adding

additional flexion through movements such as crunches is not recommended.

There is good logic to basing the majority of trunk training on movement-prevention exercises: exercises that challenge the ability to maintain a stable and controlled torso while the limbs move dynamically. If disc health is a major concern then this is likely to be a prudent policy. However, if there are no existing issues this may potentially be an excessively cautious approach which threatens to remove useful exercises. While trunk-flexion exercises may not closely represent function, they can produce a high level of targeted intensity and therefore can increase tissue capacity very effectively. Consequently it is important to explore the issues around the safety of trunk-flexion exercises.

A recent article critically evaluated the theory and research behind the sparring argument. They point out that most of the research on disc degeneration with spinal flexion is based on continuous flexing done on cadavers. These studies have involved 4,400–86,000 continuous flexions. The crucial point here is that in real life, a single session would involve far fewer sessions. Even an athlete with the 1,000 sit-up mentality would fall well short of these numbers. Of course, over the duration of a year they may accumulate this much flexion but with one crucial difference. Unlike in the cadaver, the living athlete is able to recover and regenerate in between sessions. This includes the intervertebral discs.

The ability of the discs to cope with spinal flexion thanks to inter-session repair doesn't just mean they will return to their previous health. In fact, there is evidence that spinal flexion may result in a healthier disc, due to the pump action of flexion ferrying nutrients into the disc. Of course, like any tissue there exists an optimum level. No spinal flexion and the discs may become weak. Too much and the stress will ultimately lead to trauma.

While experts will continue to disagree on this subject, it is the author's own experience that many athletes can perform spinal-flexion exercises without suffering disc issues. This is perhaps reflective of the fact that genetics are a far greater factor in disc degeneration than movement patterns. There is actually evidence of degenerative damage to discs from childhood. In summary, whenever there may be doubt it is prudent to err on the side of caution. However, coaches should not feel restricted to removing these exercises entirely, as they can form a useful addition to a programme when used appropriately.

013
goalkeepers

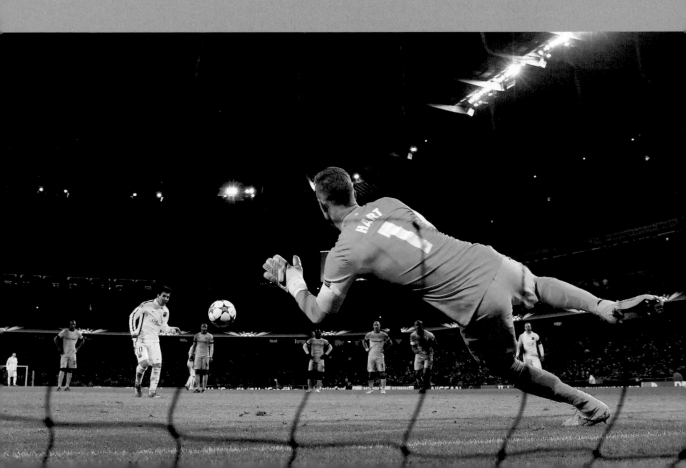

On the surface of it we have so far ignored those who stand between the sticks. The physical demands of goalkeeping differ so much from outfield play that it is understandable that many consider it a game within a game. However, while some of the specifics may differ, the fundamental principles of performance modelling, injury prevention and performance enhancement remain.

13.1 Injury Prevention

The research literature on goalkeeper injury risk is pretty sparse. However, this should not represent a major barrier to strategically planning an injury-prevention programme for goalkeepers. The difference in locomotive challenges between outfield players and goalkeepers poses different biomechanical stresses and therefore alternative injury risks. The absence of extensive sprints naturally reduces the burden on the hamstrings. However, movement is multi-directional and comprised of intermittent maximal sprints with large recoveries. Consequently, non-contact injury risk may be greater in groins, backs and knees. Of course, a large number of injuries will come from trauma associated with coming for crosses, diving at feet, etc.

If we revisit our injury-prevention model (see Chapter 5), it is likely that the players themselves and their inherent risk factors are more significant than generic position-specific concerns. Therefore a comprehensive review of injury history and an effective assessment process are critical.

Ultimately though, we must remember our first principle; the most effective method of injury-risk reduction is the planned control of the thing which will cause injury (i.e. training). Monitoring and modifying this dose will always be more potent than increasing the dose of prehab work.

Interestingly, this is an area that has been largely neglected by sports scientists. While in-depth locomotive and heart-rate data is collected on outfield players, these metrics are not particularly insightful for the goalkeeper. Very few clubs keep records of number of kicks, dives, etc., made by the goalkeepers. The technology is emerging to collect such information through algorithms which can detect these actions via the accelerometers in most movement-tracking systems. However, we surely do not need to wait for this (nor rely on it if you do not work in a club with such resources). A very simple paper scoring sheet would most likely prove highly illuminating and provide key information as to the mechanical–physical load placed on a player during a training session. Interestingly, goalkeepers are fundamentally different to outfield colleagues in that a training session will typically represent a far higher volume of work than a match. This presents some interesting questions regarding the periodisation of load through the week. The high volume of running by outfield players makes the traditional reduction in volume towards the match completely sensible. However, given that the total physical load of match play for a goalkeeper is low, and that it is chiefly a technical position (see below for more on performance factors), it could be considered prudent to maximise technical stimulus as the competition approaches. Food for thought at least.

13.2 Performance Enhancement for Goalkeepers

We have already stated that locomotive abilities represent the most obvious route to performance enhancement for outfield players. While movement is still important, there are a number of other key actions which are of primary importance for goalkeepers. If we look at the areas of training which are generally targeted we end up with three main areas of focus:

1. Leaping and jumping for saves and crosses

2. Movement, agility and mobility

3. Reactions and reflexes

Leaping and Jumping

Once upon a time, goalkeepers would run in training just as outfield players. Thankfully there has (generally) been a realisation that this is neither appropriate nor sensible. A view has started to emerge that goalkeeping is actually an explosive event hidden within a team sport. I will put my hands up and admit that I used to think that too.

Having come from a background of power athletes in track and field, I looked at what goalkeeping involves and looked at their training methods, and came to the conclusion that I could certainly make some improvements. This is possibly a very good example of why it is always better if coaches do

not immediately give in to the 'expertise' of scientists and medics. I didn't have the opportunities I would have liked initially, but I had some questions and wanted to find out more. As a result I got some of the club keepers to come and make some saves while I gathered ground reaction-force data on them. This is illustrated in Figure 13.1, below.

What this data showed conclusively was that diving to make a save, even at full stretch, is not a high-force action. This is evident from the fact that the peak force was only around 2 × body weight – similar to that of a foot strike during moderate-pace running. Even more surprising was that it can't even be considered a particularly explosive action given that the force was applied over around 350m. As surprising as these results were, on reflection they actually made a lot of sense. A dive is initiated with a falling action, with force gradually applied throughout. This is contrary to the explosive image. When we give a little more thought to the peak forces involved, these too are not so surprising. The typical average-height adult is capable of standing in the middle of a goal and diving to touch the post. Think about the photo images which are typically seen of a shot which has scored in the corner of the goal. The same image usually shows the goalkeeper covering the spot where the ball beat them, just a fraction of a second too late. Therefore it is wrong to think that more power is automatically better. The successful goalkeeper is not the one who can dive the farthest or even the quickest, but the one who is able to react first.

Armed with this information, the training strategy starts to look very different. Rather than producing players who have the strength and power qualities to produce a powerful leap, it becomes more of a

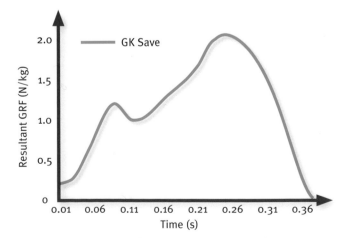

Figure 13.1 Goalkeeper's Dive GRF against other Actions

Why (some) Goalkeepers Can't Jump

There are few clubs who do not use some form of countermovement jump (CMJ) as part of their testing protocols. It is commonplace for the goalkeepers to step up to the jump mat with a degree of expectation from the tester. Sometimes this expectation is met, but often that is not the case – much to the confusion of staff and players who think goalkeepers should be the best jumpers.

The reason for this apparent anomaly is the same reason that sprinters will generally have a better CMJ than a high-jumper. A CMJ relies primarily on rapid production of large amounts of concentric force – much like the drive out the blocks of a sprinter. In contrast, the leap for a cross or even the dive for a save generally places much greater emphasis on the stretch shortening cycle (SSC) and reactive strength – much like the use of the speed coming off the bend in the high jump. Generally when a rebound is introduced to a jump challenge the goalkeepers and high-jumpers start to demonstrate the kind of jumping ability which is expected of them.

priority to equip them with the movement ability to be ready to react efficiently at all times.

If we do decide that we want to develop leaping ability in a goalkeeper it may be wise to revisit our earlier discussions around plyometrics (see Chapter 11). As we have discussed above, the leap of a goalkeeper tends to rely on elastic energy rather than the concentric power of a jump. This leads us towards plyometrics as a well-matched

training tool. However, the view that sufficient plyometric volume may be accumulated in normal training seems particularly pertinent in the case of the goalkeeper. Training typically involves large volumes of highly specific jump-type activity. Therefore adding to this volume is unlikely to achieve significant augmentation of performance and may risk drifting towards excessive load. Given the lessons we have learned from Prue Cormie regarding the balance of strength and power training, it may be a more effective approach to use S&C sessions to develop force-production ability (i.e. strength) and treat on-pitch work as special preparatory work.

S&C coaches may wish to use ballistic jumps as a form of specific preparatory work within the gym. These can be a highly effective tool for the expression and development of explosive power. There is an interesting paradox here though, as optimal jumping technique ≠ optimal save technique. Whatever the exercise, when jumping for power it is crucial that movements are performed with a proximo–distal kinetic chain, in plain English – hips, knees and ankles extend in that order. This means keeping a solid, flat-foot contact on the floor as long as possible in order to maximise transfer of force down from the powerful hips and knees. Conversely, when we watch goalkeepers move they tend to stay on the balls of their feet. This is logical as it allows careful movement of the feet to achieve optimal positioning and balance. While some capacity for force generation is lost, as we have seen, this is unlikely to be a limiting factor. So, when coaching jump skills in the gym it is important that we retain an awareness that the technical cues we are giving in the gym may differ from those given by the goalkeeping coach. Making both the coach and player aware of this may be a smart move to avoid conflict and potential negative transfer from your coaching.

Goalkeeping – It's all in the ankles?

During the writing of this book, I recently paid a visit to watch some tae kwon do fighters train. Much like goalkeepers, these fighters are constantly 'on their toes', ready to either launch a kicking attack, plant for a punch or move to elude an opponent's attack. These athletes place a huge emphasis in training on ankle stability and have some excellent plyometric drills and skills. On watching them it struck me how this transfers to goalkeeping. By maintaining a stable ankle the 'keeper is able to stay mobile and ready to move by avoiding being caught flat footed, but also has a firm base to push off so that their dive is not dampened by energy leaks at the ankle.'

I have not had the chance at the time of writing to measure ankle stability in goalkeepers during typical play, or to specifically target ankle stability for performance enhancement. My suspicion though is that this may be one of the most effective routes to physical performance enhancement. Watch this space ...

Movement, Agility and Mobility

Having learnt that diving for saves is not dependent on huge expressions of power, our attentions shift towards the ability to be well positioned to execute the save as quickly as possible. When I was reflecting on the results of my force investigations I discussed them with highly experienced and knowledgeable goalkeeping coach at the club, Dean Kiely, who gave me the following insightful quote:

'...you are constantly adjusting to correct your own movement mistakes.'

By this he meant that every time something changes in the 'picture' in front of you, it changes what your ideal position should be. Therefore good movement is a constant process of subtle adjustments. With this in mind, the dramatic diving save is almost the last resort. When movement is optimal, a goalkeeper is able to adjust their feet and collect the ball much more comfortably. This is similar to the famous Paulo Maldini quote that defenders should not have to make a tackle or dirty their shorts – they simply need to read the game better.

This raises the obvious question of the role of S&C in movement development, as the cognitive ability to read the game is clearly paramount. This alone is a valuable realisation, as sometimes what we don't do is as important as the things we do. Essentially good movement can be supported by strength, mobility and control to enable good physical literacy, so that each movement challenge can be met with an appropriate response. Rather than attempt to recreate or plan for every possible eventuality, it is more practical to provide players with a good foundation of functional movement, which should be considered the start point for any athletic development programme.

Improving Reactions

Sports manufacturers have produced a variety of training aids which are intended to help improve reaction times. Tools such as reaction balls and reaction walls work on the basis of forcing the player to respond to unpredictable stimuli, in the hope that this will generically improve reaction time. It is worth taking a step back though and looking at exactly what has to happen in order for

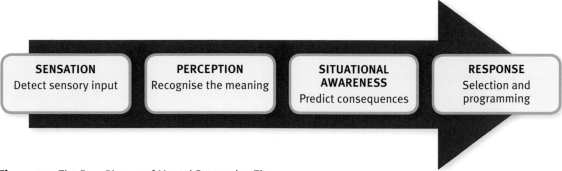

SENSATION
Detect sensory input

PERCEPTION
Recognise the meaning

SITUATIONAL AWARENESS
Predict consequences

RESPONSE
Selection and programming

Figure 13.2 The Four Phases of Mental Processing Time

a player to produce a reaction (to anything). This is illustrated in Figure 13.2.

The process begins with **sensory input** (generally visual in this case). The visual cues which trigger a response differ between experts and novices. Novice goalkeepers will often not react until the ball is in flight following a shot, whereas experts are able to take much earlier cues such as the movement of the hips of a striker. Once these cues have been detected we move into **perception**. For example, having noticed a shift in weight in the striker, the goalkeeper recognises this is likely to lead to a shot. The consequences of this need to be predicted during the **situational awareness** phase. Finally, having interpreted all of the external information the goalkeeper can formulate an appropriate **response** and, in lay terms, the mind can tell the body what it needs to do. Of course, all of these processes happen incredibly quickly and subconsciously, but each is critical. This sequence of mental processing is the underpinning engineering of what we generally call 'reactions'. This is then followed by the reflexes (i.e. how quickly you can action the response).

This reaction time is undoubtedly trainable. However, the training effect comes from familiarity and recognition of cues and associated responses. Therefore it is highly situation-specific. This is bad news for the toy manufacturers as there is no carry-over between reacting to a non-specific stimulus such as a randomly bouncing ball or flashing lights going off. What may surprise many is that the actual reflex time (i.e. the time between deciding what to do and actioning it) is no different between elite sportsmen and novices.

So, it seems that rather than directing our efforts towards improving reflexes in goalkeepers, we may be more effective in seeking to develop reaction times and ability to recognise specific visual cues. The natural and probably most effective method of achieving this is to expose the player to as many learning opportunities as possible through realistic training scenarios (i.e. realistic game play rather than static shots in an artificial manner). This is of course the realm of the coaching staff rather than being an S&C concern. The exception to this may come during a period of rehabilitation from injury. Following a medium- to long-term lay-off it is common for goalkeepers to feel they need several training sessions to 'get their eye back in'. This can lead to a delayed return to match availability. Consequently there is value to be added if we can accelerate this process. There are now tools available, such as those used in the GSK Human Performance Lab, which can help to assess and train reactions to visual stimuli in a specific manner without the physical act taking place. This approach uses video clips, frozen at key time points, to assess and develop a player's ability to recognise specific cues. This can potentially serve as an effective method of maintaining technical ability during rehab or augmenting technical exposure when physical tolerance has become the limiting factor in training time.

Practical Goalkeeper Training

The No. 1 position is no different to any other player, in that S&C prescription should be tailored to specific playing profile and physical characteristics of the individual. However, while there are still obvious differences in how they play the game, the playing profile clearly differs less between goalkeepers than it does between outfield players. On that basis the broad guidelines given in Table 13.1 serve as a potential starting point for a goalkeeping S&C framework.

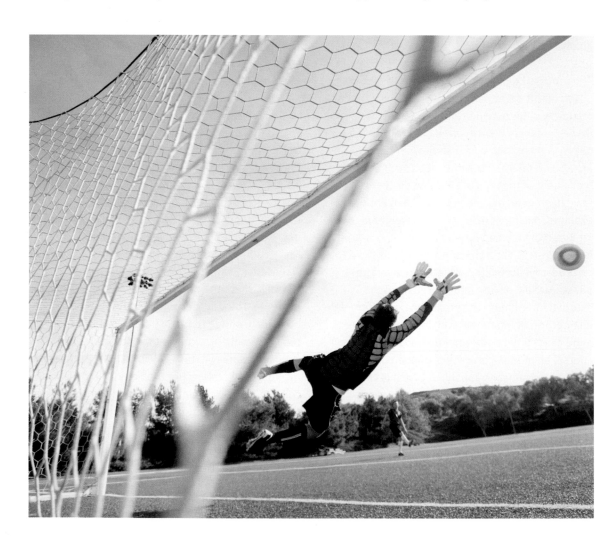

Table 13.1	Example S&C Focus Areas for Goalkeepers	
Focus	**Rationale**	**Examples**
Maximum strength	To enhance force production and complement specific jump work in training	Bilateral strength lifts, such as back and front squat
Concentric power	To support short accelerations and leaps from a static position	Ballistic jumping exercises and loaded explosive exercises such as jump squats
High-load trunk work	To provide protection against the need to tolerate high forces through the trunk during game play	May include whole-body resistance exercises such as squats, but also trunk-specific work with a focus on isometric control against multi-directional forces
Low-threshold trunk work	Important for optimal spinal stabilisation and the avoidance of reliance on superior musculature	Pilates-type activities such as bird-dogs and dead bugs, with an emphasis on control
Thoracic mobility	Important for reducing the burden on the shoulders and lumbar spine	Mobilising techniques such as foam rollers and yoga/Pilates through flexion, extension, lateral flexion and rotation
Low level plyometrics	To ensure optimal alignment on landings and CoD to avoid movement dysfunctions	Controlled unilateral landing drills such as hop-stick
Multi-directional movement patterns	To develop strength through range and reflect the non-linear nature of goalkeeper movement	Lunge patterns such as the clock lunge and side step-ups

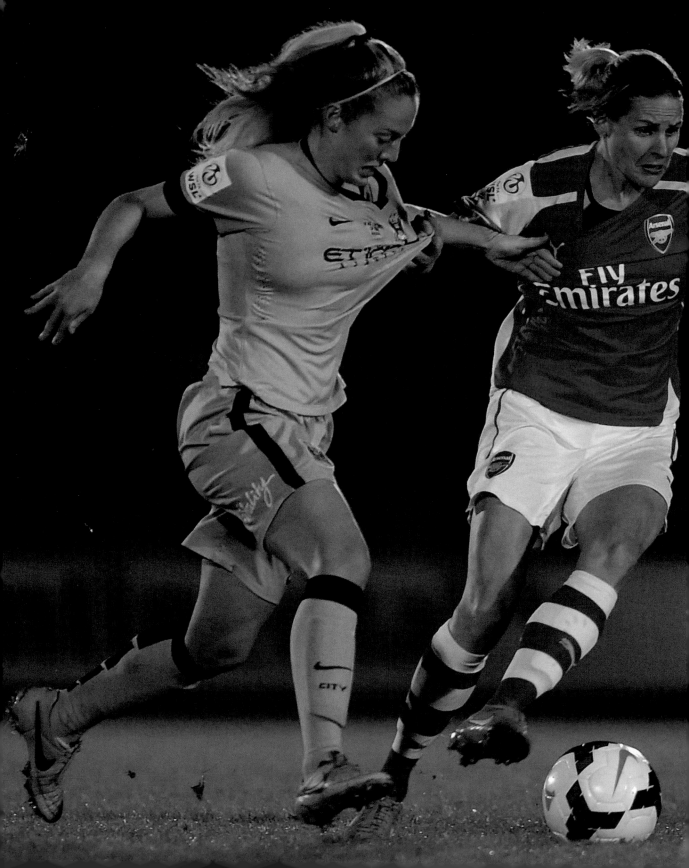

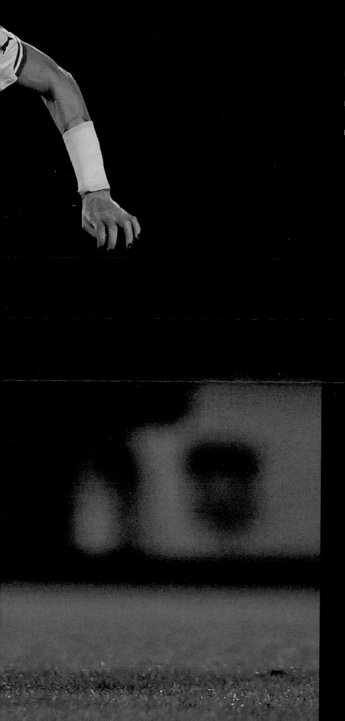

part 4

applied lessons

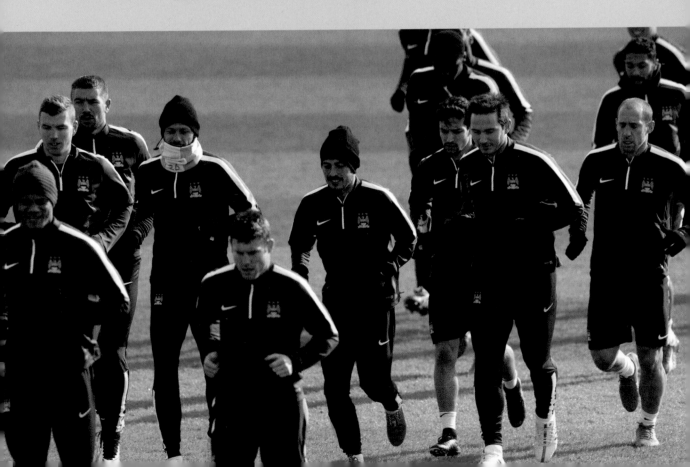

014
programming and planning

14.1 Measurement of Training

It is a fundamental requirement of all training that we are able to measure what we do. Without this ability we cannot make the subtle and precise changes needed to conform with the principles of overload and progression.

The most common method of measuring gym training is **volume load** (VL). This is simply calculated by multiplying the volume (sets × reps) by the weight lifted (intensity). For example, 3 sets of 10 reps at 20kg give a VL of 600kg (3 × 10 × 20). The steady, week-on-week, month-on-month progress which is seen in resistance training relies heavily on our ability to make and measure small adjustments to a training load.

Unfortunately, monitoring of training intensity is often not quite as simple when it comes to conditioning work, as many exercises do not use any additional load. This means that our measure of intensity has been removed. The measure of volume is also less clear, as many conditioning exercises, particularly around the trunk, are focused on prevention of unwanted movement and so there are often no distinct repetitions performed, as a position is held for a period of time. For these isometric exercises our measure of volume, i.e. reps, has also now been lost. This can make comparisons between exercises difficult. For example, how many crunches are equal to a 30-second plank hold? All of these factors contribute to the common situation whereby conditioning levels tend to plateau quickly and remain relatively static. This is hardly surprising when we consider how our measures of volume and intensity have been compromised, and in turn our precision in overloading and progressing exercise prescription.

One solution to the issue of measuring volume may be that, rather than counting reps, we can measure all volume in terms of time, or more specifically, time under tension (TUT). This allows us to compare between isometric and dynamic training. If exercises are set according to time rather than reps it can also have a beneficial effect on quality of technique. If players are not chasing a fixed number and trying to rush, they will often be more deliberate and controlled in their performance. Of course, movement must be constant otherwise we will only have accumulated time rather than TUT.

The issue of defining the intensity of an exercise is somewhat harder. Ultimately I do not believe there is a perfect system, as the range of exercises used in conditioning mean that we are not comparing like with like. However, a method which I have found to provide a much greater structure and bridge the gap needed to allow better programming precision is to simply assign arbitrary intensity values to the range of conditioning exercises which I prescribe. These values are not supported by scientific evidence, but are simply the product of coach experience of having performed and

Table 14.1	Example Conditioning-Intensity Classification System
Movement Type	**Intensity Value**
Low level/motor control	1
Low-intensity isolation work	2–3
High-intensity isolation work	4–5
Whole-body barbell exercises	6–7
Eccentrics	8–10

prescribed the exercises and knowing how they compare. Theoretically it may be possible to use EMG to compare muscle-activation levels across key exercises. However, the scale of such a task is enormous and most likely unnecessary.

When taking such an approach it is important that the scoring criteria and range are given close consideration. The subjective and abstract nature of this method of measuring intensity means that such systems are likely to vary considerably between coaches. However, I have illustrated the systems I have used below as an example. Table 14.1 on the previous page outlines the scoring criteria used to rank exercises.

By defining clear categories for exercise intensities in this way it is relatively easy to be consistent when assigning intensity scores to new exercises. As a note of caution, it may be necessary to increase the score assigned to high-intensity lifts, in order to avoid a bias towards high volumes of low-intensity work. The tables (14.2–14.5) below provide real-life examples of this system being applied to a range of typical conditioning challenges, namely: glutes, calves, hamstrings and the trunk.

Table 14.2	Glute-Conditioning Challenges					
Exercise	**Level**					
	1	**2**	**3**	**4**	**5**	**6**
Hurdles	Standard					
A-March	Standard					
Superman	Standard					
Band Walks			Standard			
Fire Hydrants		BW	Ankle			
Clam Shells		BW	Resisted			
Hip Hitch		BW	DB			
Bench Hip Raise		BW	Resisted			
SL Bench Hip Raise			BW	Resisted		
Glute Bridge		BW	20kg	Manual	40+kg	
SL Glute Bridge			BW	20kg	Manual	
Hip Dominant Squat						Loaded

Note: BW = body weight, DB = dumbbell, SL = single leg

Table 14.3	Calf-Conditioning Challenges				
Exercise	**Level**				
	1	**2**	**3**	**4**	**5**
Proprioception & Balance	Various				
Sand Work		Various			
Rebound Ankle Jumps		Standard			
Single Leg Rebound Ankle Jumps			Standard		
Seated Calf Raise		BW	Barbell		
Calf Raise		BW	Kettlebell		
Single Leg Calf Raise			BW	Kettlebell	Barbell

Note: BW = body weight

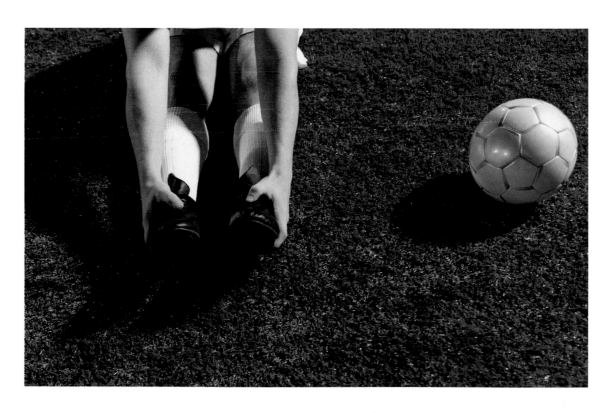

Table 14.4	Hamstring-Conditioning Challenges								
Exercise	**Level**								
	1	2	3	4	5	6	7	8	9
Fold & Extend	Standard								
C-Drill		Standard							
Flutters		Standard							
Reactive		Standard							
Hamstring Bridge		BW	PB						
SL Hamstring Bridge				BW	PB				
Swiss Ball Curls			Bilateral	Unilateral					
Sled Tow			⟵20kg	⟶20kg					
Glute-Ham Raise			Standard	Weighted		SL			
Hamstring Curls			Light	Med	Heavy			Ecc (mod)	Ecc (hard)
Scooter Pulls			Standard						
Good Mornings			SL	Med	Heavy				
RDL					Light	Moderate	Heavy		
Nordics								Standard	High Qual

Note: BW = body weight, PB = power bag, Ecc = eccentric, SL = single leg

Table 14.5	Trunk-Conditioning Challenges				
Exercise	**Level**				
	1	**2**	**3**	**4**	**5**
Pelvic Rolls		Standard			
Dead Bugs		Standard	Weighted	Isometric	
Aleknas		BW	5–10kg	10kg+	
Woodchops		Light	Heavy		
Side Bends		0–5kg	6–10kg		
Pavlov Press			Standard		
Swiss Ball Plank			Standard		
Double Leg Lower			Standard		
Front Plank			Basic	3-point	Weighted
Side Plank			Basic	Leg lifts	Resisted
Deep Press-Ups			Basic	Weighted	
Back Extension Holds			Basic	Arms out	
Suitcase Deadlift			Light	Heavy	
V-Sits				Standard	
Roll Outs				Standard	
Hanging Leg Raises				Standard	
Candle Sticks				Partial	Full

14.2 Periodisation

Macro-cycles

Periodisation in football can be a complex and difficult topic. At a most basic level, simply defining priority periods within the calendar is a challenge. Within a league structure all games are of equal points value, and the level of opposition is randomly distributed throughout the season. A handful of the most successful clubs in the Premier League are able to go into a season with good confidence that they expect to be competing for honours in most of the major competitions towards the end of the season. In competitions with a knock-out format, the level of competition should, at least in theory, get progressively harder through the rounds. Therefore there is merit in an end-of-season peaking model. At other clubs for whom survival is success, they may take the view that they would like to get as many points as quickly as possible to secure safety.

In reality though, the approach to S&C in football may be best positioned a step back from this debate. If our first goal is injury prevention then this is something which should be optimised as a constant rather than travelling through peaks and troughs. Unlike the traditional view of performance enhancement whereby a peak performance level is achieved for a brief but unsustainable period, robustness should sit at an optimum level throughout. Perhaps the only caveat to that would be that during times of intense competition demands there may be a need for increased focus on maintaining health. In this situation the S&C coach is faced with a difficult balance between providing a protective effect and the risk of adding to an already large physical load. As the graph in Figure 14.1 below demonstrates, there is a strong trend towards injury rates reducing as the season progresses. This would suggest that players return from the summer ill-prepared for the high volumes of training during pre-season and are still in the process of adapting to training and competition demands for several months into a competitive season. It would suggest that a review of off-season conditioning and pre-season training may be warranted.

The need to modulate performance enhancement work through the season is very much dependent on the training level of the player. As we have discussed previously, many players will be able to make genuine performance gains through improved movement quality and athleticism, rather than through gains in strength and power. For these players the physical demands of the work are likely to be low, and so progression can be made in an ongoing manner independent of the seasonal priority. Players who are engaged in high-intensity strength and power work may require intelligent modulation of load through the season. This will in part involve the management of fatigue through the meso- and micro-cycles (see below). On a macro-scale then, naturally the

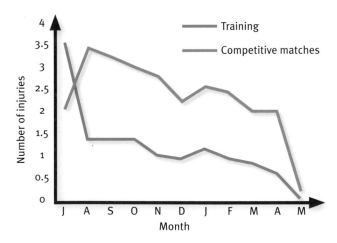

Figure 14.1 Mean Monthly Injury Rates in Professional Football
Source: Hawkins et al. (2001)

planning must be matched to the pattern of the season identified by coaching staff and on-field conditioners. As we've seen, this is very much on a club-by-club basis. However, one common approach which seems based on good logic splits the season broadly into three sections of similar duration. The first is treated as a **development** phase whereby training gains are still being made during the competitive calendar. This is a reasonable assertion given the relatively brief pre-season period. The middle section of the season is regarded as **maintenance**. Here the aim is to achieve a balance between sufficient load to maintain previous gains while managing fatigue. Finally, the season ends with a **freshness** focus. By this stage the ongoing build-up of games through the first two-thirds of the season means that players will be suffering from residual fatigue. The point at which training gains can be made has been lost and therefore recovery from competition is primary.

The view is often taken that the pre-season period can be used as general preparation, with this window being regarded as the only real opportunity to make strength gains. This is based on the assumption that the absence of competitive gains makes fatigue from the gym a more acceptable side-effect. It also comes from the concept that it is impossible to make strength gains in-season. However, if we return to the injury profile shown above in Figure 14.1, it would appear that players generally do not cope well with pre-season training loads. Several weeks of very minimal training through the restorative summer are swiftly followed by enormous increases in volume. This often includes double sessions with volume higher than at any point during the season. Consequently, adding to this volume with large volumes of strength training may not be prudent. With regard to the concept that strength gains

cannot be made in season, this clearly does not add up when we consider the typical strength profile of a player. Of course, the conflicting demands on the body of football training and strength training mean that it would be impossible for an individual to reach their full genetic potential in the gym. However, it absolutely does not mean that moderate levels of strength cannot be improved upon. The Glasgow Warriors S&C coach, Stuart Yule, has discussed the need to continually improve strength qualities in his players through the season. If that is achievable in a strength-trained population of elite rugby league players, it is certainly possible in professional football.

Meso-cycles

The structure of the meso-cycles within a periodised football S&C programme is to some extent simply a matter of coach philosophy and preference. Many players will have only limited experience of strength-training regimes. Therefore the so-called 'novice effect' is likely to be present, whereby they improve regardless of the system the coach chooses to implement. All training stimulus is novel to them, and so adaptation is almost inevitable. As players grow in training age though, the need for intelligently structured and well-planned programmes becomes more important.

Given that football is not a single or even double-peak sport, block periodisation is unlikely to be appropriate. Instead some form of conjugate or mixed-methods programme is perhaps best matched to the demands of a season and the opportunity to enhance several qualities simultaneously. The optimal progression of load is also highly individual. Coaches may prefer an undulating or linear method, but either can be successful. What is arguably more important is that suitable monitoring processes are in place to enable evidence-based reflection, and to provide the coach with insight into readiness to train and adaptation to training. The concept of a 'test week' at the end of a training block has fallen out of favour in recent years. This is reflection of the fact that the human body is complex and hard to predict. While a training programme on paper may neatly illustrate how a player will peak at week 6, this is often not the case in real life. Therefore simple monitoring in training gives a much clearer picture of how the player has responded over the course of the training. Typical examples include using a switch mat to measure jump heights, or a linear encoder to assess bar velocity. These have the added value of providing highly motivational feedback to a player and enhancing their effort and focus.

Micro-cycles

The planning of the micro-cycle is naturally dependent on the pattern and frequency of competitive fixtures. Clearly a model which suits a Saturday-to-Saturday schedule does not work if there is also a mid-week fixture. In the latter example, progressive training becomes extremely challenging as players are most likely to simply play, recover, play. If there are seven days between fixtures, then a schedule which places the greatest training load in the middle of the week makes most sense. This allows for recovery from the previous match, but without impacting on the following match.

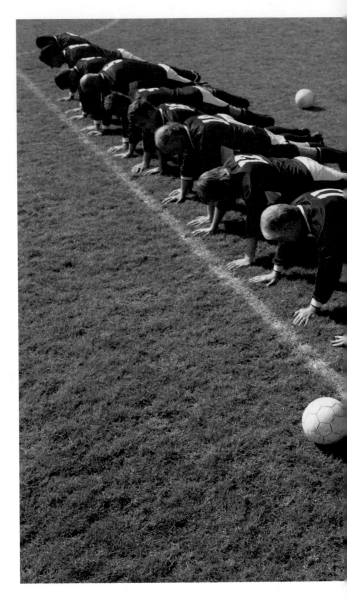

The use of resistance training as a priming tool prior to a match may have some potential to enhance performance. This involves the use of a low-volume, high-quality training stimulus in a window of anywhere between 1 and 24 hours prior to competition in order to gain a short-term hormonal or neuromuscular adaptation. This might come in the form of a short resistance-training session, some sprints or some jumps. This type of tool is probably somewhat underused in football. Typically this is due to a fear of leaving residual fatigue in a player and impairing, rather than enhancing, performance. As a result, resistance-training based priming sessions are likely to be a hard sell. When they are used the player should of

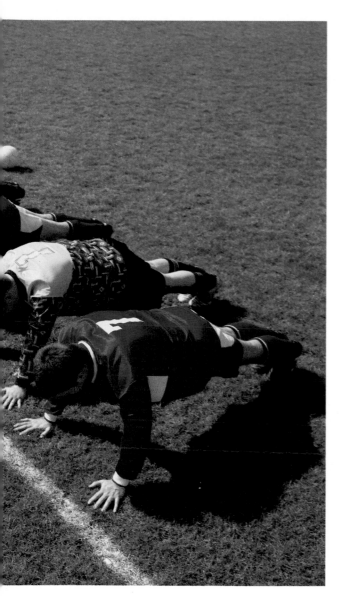

The structure of the training day raises a number of questions around concurrent training, or the interference effect. It has long been established that strength training and endurance training (on-pitch football in this case) performed in close proximity can blunt the adaptation of each other. Recently a lot of attention has been placed on how best to sequence these two types of training stimulus in order to achieve the best outcome. Two opposing schools of thought exist in this debate. The first would suggest that the endurance work should follow the strength work to avoid the negative impact of fatigue on the neuromuscular performance in the gym. This seems logical. However, an opposing viewpoint gives consideration to the cell signalling which underpins adaptation to training. Given that an endurance session will 'shut-down' the pathways (MToR) which trigger strength adaptations, then the strength session should be performed last. At present there is not enough evidence to say definitively that either of these viewpoints is 100% correct. Perhaps though this is rather convenient. Players typically have a firm view as to whether they like to come to the gym before or after training. The nature of the session should also influence the S&C coach's decision as to when to schedule it. If the gym work planned is hard and fatiguing, then it would be unwise to place it immediately before pitch work. This is likely to increase the risk of injury and impact on the quality of the football session – neither of which is good for the job security of an S&C coach. In an ideal world, sessions would be placed as far apart as possible. This is often not practical though, as professional football clubs frequently operate with a single training window per day. The exceptions to this come in pre-season and when a player is injured. During these times the intelligent spacing and sequencing of sessions may help to enhance and optimise the adaptations that follow.

course be highly accustomed to the exercise choices, to avoid an adverse reaction to a novel stimulus. Sprints and jumps may be a more palatable option for many. This may also provide a psychological boost as the player can feel quick and explosive and takes confidence in his ability into the match.

015
practical tools

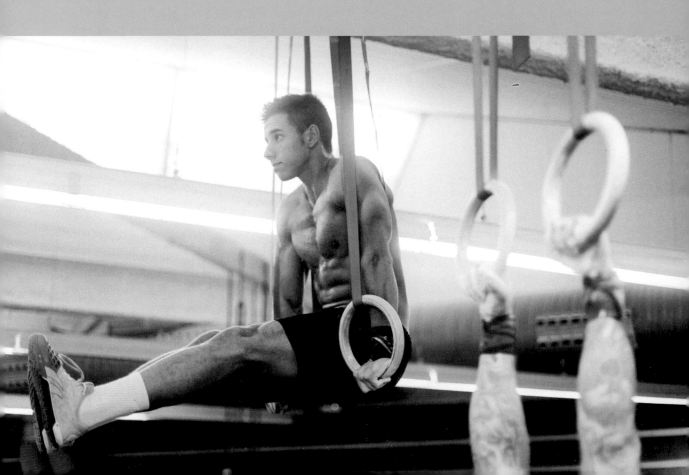

The aim throughout this book has very much been to 'teach a man to fish' rather than 'give a man a fish'. That is to say, if an S&C coach understands clearly the adaptations that they are seeking and the characteristics of exercises that will achieve them, then selecting those exercises becomes a very simple process. This is far more empowering than following a recipe-type of approach. Consequently the aim of this chapter is to reiterate some of the key principles behind injury prevention and performance enhancement, and to provide some example practical tools which illustrate the points made and potentially serve as a starting point for coaches exploring a new approach.

Rather than grouping exercises in terms of muscles, we will categorise exercises in terms of movements and the outcome to which they are best suited, e.g. explosive movements, etc. The technique for many of these, such as Olympic lifts and whole-body barbell lifts, is underpinned by a good depth of technical understanding. Therefore exercises are cited as examples, with background given to the adaptation and classification of an exercise rather than an instructional guide to technical performance. Texts such as *Starting Strength* provide an excellent overview of the technical performance of many of these movements, particularly barbell strength exercises. However, books should not be the sole source of information for such activity, and novice coaches should seek assistance from experienced practitioners who can provide feedback where a book cannot.

15.1 Athleticism and Fundamental Movements

If an S&C programme achieves nothing other than giving a player a greater foundation for athleticism and fundamental movements, it can still be considered successful. Great gains in our headline goals of injury prevention and performance enhancement can be made through this route alone.

The Squat

The squat is arguably the king of exercises. It is often the first movement evaluated in a functional screen, and is a staple in strength-training programmes. It demands range of movement through the hips, knees and ankles, and demands stability in these joints at the same time. It provides an ideal challenge for increasing force production in the limbs and force tolerance through the trunk. The fact that all of these qualities are trained in concert means that the transfer to general athleticism is far more natural than if they were developed in isolation. As a bilateral lift, stability is not challenged as much as during single-leg movements. Therefore, in terms of quality of movement, developing mobility and range of movement is where the squat is most effective. Consequently, gains in this area, as demonstrated by moving towards a full-depth squat, are just as valid as adding load to the bar. It is important to state that what constitutes full depth will vary significantly between players. A key factor in this is the structure of the hip joint itself. It is a big mistake to try to guide all players towards a uniform depth of squats, which will lead to failure and possible injury.

Of course, the squat is more a family of exercises rather than a single exercise. There are seemingly endless variations on a theme including Zercher squats, goblet squats, sumo squats, and many more. Fundamentally though there are three main forms of the exercise, namely: back squat, front squat and the overhead squat.

Contrary to popular belief, muscle activation levels in the hip and knee extensors do not appear to differ significantly between the front

153

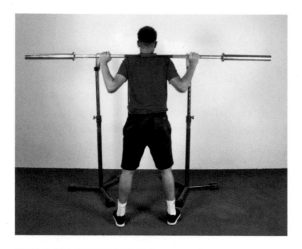

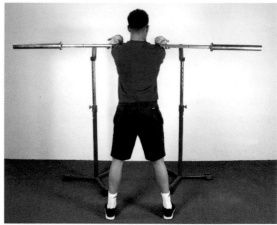

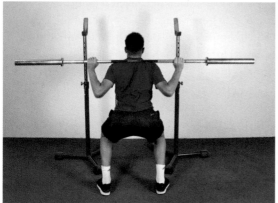

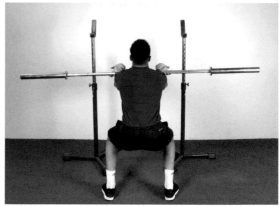

Back Squat

Front Squat

and back squat. The back squat is often the starting point for coaching a squatting movement to a player. Holding the bar across the shoulders is generally more comfortable than the front-squat position for many beginners due to a lack of flexibility in the lats and wrists. I believe it is important that players learn to hold a back-squat position without the use of a so-called 'sissy pad'. Even the leanest individual should be able to retract their shoulders sufficiently to allow the bar to sit comfortably on the trapezius. The use of a pad gives the player 'permission' to neglect this important aspect of posture and therefore

compromise their technique. Typically players will achieve greater loadings with a back squat over a front squat (although this should not be confused with greater muscular effort). However, the front-bar position is often favourable for individuals with long femurs who find an appropriate trunk angle hard to achieve in the back position. For coaches who wish to utilise the power clean as a training tool, the front squat holds the added benefit of helping to develop strength in the catch position. There are numerous internet coach debates over whether back squats represent too much of a threat to back health, and should be replaced by front squats exclusively, or even just single-leg options. This ignores our ability as coaches to evaluate the suitability of a lift on an individual basis. Ultimately, good coaching involves selecting the correct lift according to a player's own anthropometrics and training needs. This should continue into the subtle nuances of the lift including depth, foot position, etc.

It is extremely common for squat depth in footballers to be limited by a lack of mobility in their ankles. The use of proper weightlifting shoes alleviates this problem somewhat, due to the small heel raise which is incorporated into the shoe. If this is insufficient then small discs can be placed underneath the heels to allow the movement to be performed properly. It is critical that this is only used as a short-term solution, though. The player must be cued to sit back through their heels and press them into the plates. If this is followed then the discs can quickly be reduced and removed and the player will have gained valuable range through their ankles. However, failure to distribute the weight through the foot correctly will mean that mobility at the ankle is not challenged, and will not progress.

If the squat in general is considered one of the most effective single tools for developing athleticism, the overhead squat is the godfather. The additional challenge to the upper body through thoracic and shoulder mobility also adds to the demands throughout the body due to the influence of myofascial slings. When it comes to global mobility, there is nowhere to hide in the overhead squat. The absolute load, i.e. the weight on the bar, will be lower than in a back or front squat. However, what is lost in general strength stimulus is compensated by a high level of activity required to maintain posture and control throughout the movement. Some would term this

'functional strength', although the obvious counter that holding a barbell above your head and squatting represents practically no sporting task (except the snatch lift) makes this term somewhat redundant. As a note of caution, a great many players do not walk into the gym possessing sufficient thoracic mobility to perform this movement correctly. Naturally, this can be developed, and the overhead squat can be a good means of identifying the deficit. However, the widespread prescription of overhead squats without compromise is likely to lead to several issues and bad techniques. Most commonly you

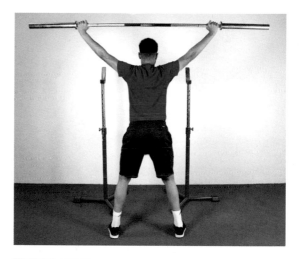

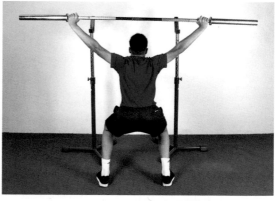

Overhead Squat

will see players attempting to perform the lift with their spine almost vertical, and feeling back pain as a result of the effort.

Finally, the dead lift can also be classed as being in the squatting family. The benefits to athleticism are equally valid with this lift. The most important distinction comes from the fact that the dead lift is classified as a pull rather than a press like the squat. This means that it is an extension-dominant movement, and therefore the posterior

musculature, particularly the hamstrings, play a greater role in generating force. This makes the lift appealing in a football squad as we seek to redress the natural balance and overcome the dominance of the quads that is typically seen in players. It is vital that technique is not compromised in the dead lift in order to overcome excessive loads. This is a salient point as technical failure generally comes before absolute failure. If back health is a concern then the load on the lumbar spine can be reduced through the use of trap bar deadlifts (below). It is also worth pointing out that the starting height of the bar, as determined by the size of the plates used, is entirely arbitrary. That is to say, this is not some cleverly calculated height that all humans should be able to reach. If the bar needs to be raised to enable the player to hold good form and feel strong, then the coach should not hesitate in doing so. It is then possible over time to gradually reduce this height and gain mobility, but not at the cost of safety or form.

Single-Leg Movements

As we have seen, the impact of bilateral lifts on movement quality is biased towards mobility over stability. The reverse is true during unilateral, or single-leg, lifts. Of course, the definition of a single-leg lift isn't strictly accurate as many, such as the split squat or the Bulgarian squat, involve two points of contact with the ground throughout the movement. The degree to which the base of support is spread across two points ultimately determines how great the stability challenge faced will be. For example, a split squat allows both feet to stay in contact with the ground throughout the movement, therefore the stability required is relatively low. On the other hand, the movement during a step-up takes place primarily on one leg, which is highly flexed. Consequently the demands required to hold form are much greater.

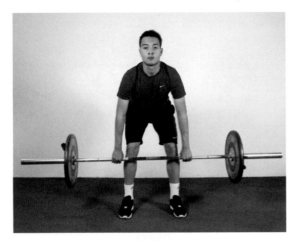

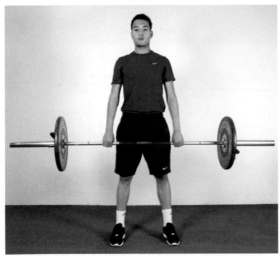

Dead Lift

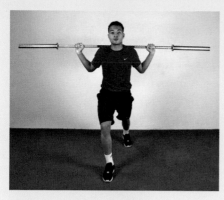

Split Squat

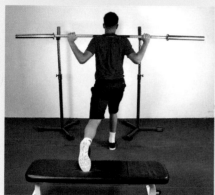
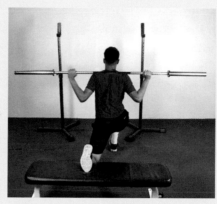

Bulgarian Squat

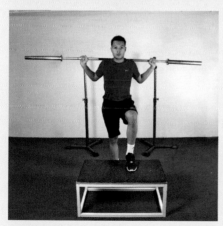
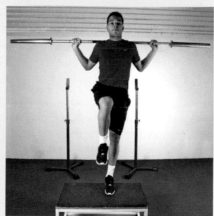

Box Step-Up

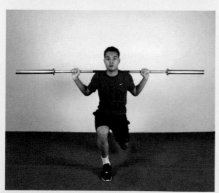

Lunge

A continuum of stable to unstable classic unilateral lifts is illustrated in Figure 15.1.

As we can see, this continuum of exercises moves from a constant bilateral support (split squat), through to a compromised bilateral support (Bulgarian squat). We then move onto a single base of support (step-up) and finally to an impact absorbing support (lunge). This final exercise, the lunge, is a particularly useful tool in a multi-directional sport such as football as it can be manipulated to become multiplanar. The classic forward lunge is actually a load-acceptance exercise as the lead leg is primarily required to control forces on landing. A reverse lunge changes the emphasis to an effective pulling movement through the posterior chain (glutes and hamstrings). Finally, the lateral lunge is excellent for challenging the lower body through a movement plane which is often neglected in gym training. Of course, when the stability challenge is high, the capacity to load a lift becomes reduced. Coaches should consider these factors, among others, when selecting the lift they prescribe.

Presses and Pulls

While the general perception of squatting movements has moved to a more enlightened view than simply 'leg weights', the understanding of many upper-body movements still often lags behind somewhat. When good, whole-body choices are used these can help to develop movement quality around the shoulder girdle and, critically, lumbo–pelvic control while transferring forces across the trunk.

If we take the humble press-up as an example, the player is required to maintain perfect form and lumbar stability through the trunk while pressing throughout the movement, which requires deep abdominal strength and control. If we were to view

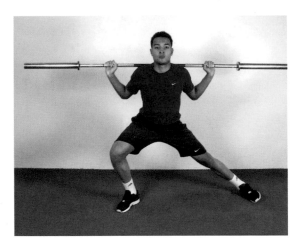

Lateral Lunge

this from the narrow mindset of press-ups being a 'chest exercise', then we are less likely to be concerned with control through the abdomen and more focused on achieving a burn in the pecs and pushing through to failure. This shows how two coaches can prescribe the same exercise, but the thinking and understanding behind the prescription can lead to very different outcomes.

If we are to look at pulling movements, the classic pull-up also presents some appealing athletic challenges for the S&C coach to utilise. Before any movement has occurred, simply hanging while keeping the ribcage down and the scapulae set may prove difficult for many (including those who can smash out decent numbers of ugly repetitions). Just as with press-ups, once the movement starts it is then important to keep the spine in a neutral position throughout, rather than going into full extension and thus failing to stabilise anteriorly. If we consider that this locking into extension strategy is the one taken by many players during sprint running, and subsequently increases the risk of injury such as a pars fracture in the lumbar spine, then clearly form is more important than reps.

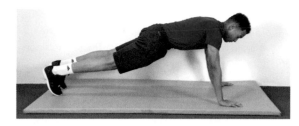

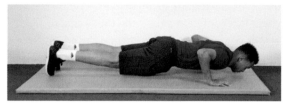

Press-Ups

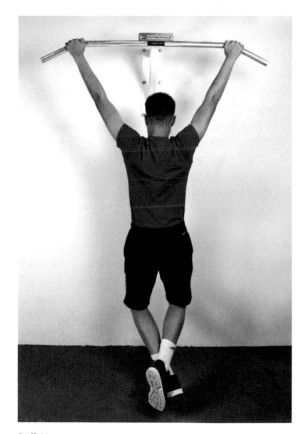

Pull-Ups

All of the above, from back squats to press-ups, are examples of viewing exercises primarily as tools to enhance movement abilities rather than simply an increase in force production or muscle mass. Hopefully this illustrates that it is not what you do but how you do it. The examples we have chosen are some of those most commonly seen in the gym and are particularly effective due to their whole-body nature. However, this same philosophy can be extended to all forms of training. This no-compromise approach to technique is suggested on the basis that we are attempting to build athletes, rather than a fussy approach or a desire to use athletes as a shop window for your technical knowledge. The key to successfully implementing this type of philosophy is to start with excellent technique (if you can't attain it, strip the exercise back to an easier level). This method of starting with technical excellence and then adding capacity undoubtedly works far better than the reverse.

15.2 Performance Qualities – Upgrading the Engine

Having developed an excellent base of movement quality there inevitably comes a point where we want to start to increase a player's capacity to produce, reduce and redirect force. As we've already stated, the most effective strength and power exercises are those in which the individual player feels able to produce the appropriate levels of force. However, that is not to ignore the fact that the various options available each carry their own relative merits and specific characteristics which lend themselves to particular aspects of strength.

15.3 General Strength Training

The starting point may simply be to develop 'general strength'. The use of the exercises such as the squat patterns which we have initially used to develop athletic movement qualities can now start to be loaded up to provide more of a strength stimulus. The reason this is described as general strength is that the physical adaption is likely to be a general upshift of the force–velocity curve. That is to say, the player will become stronger through a movement in a uniform pattern, particularly if there is a good intent to move the bar explosively. If this is not the case then there may be a bias towards maximum strength rather than explosive elements such as rate of force

development. The characteristics of the exercise can be manipulated to change this through the use of tools such as bands and chains. These increase the downward vertical load towards the end of the lift, thus reducing the natural deceleration which occurs towards the end of non-explosive lifts such as squats and dead lifts. The box squat can also be useful in this regard, as the player is required to come to a complete pause and thus remove any elastic contribution to the upward thrust.

Jump Squats

The jump squat is perhaps the most simple and natural way in which an S&C coach can achieve a loaded triple-extension movement (of hips, knees and ankles) with a group of players. The movement requires little coaching, and the small depth of descent means that mobility and stability should not become limiting factors. Typically the lift is performed as essentially a countermovement jump with a bar across the shoulders. This has the advantage of taking a natural action rather than training a new movement, and so a great deal of the player's attention can be placed upon effort. The use of feedback in the form of jump height from a jump mat or similar undoubtedly has a positive impact on effort, and I would recommend its use whenever possible.

Although the jump squat does feature a stretch-shortening cycle, the contribution of elastic energy to power production is relatively small. Therefore this movement transfers very well to the concentric power, which is so important for accelerations. Power outputs in the region of 4,000–5,000 watts have been seen in team sports players, illustrating the effectiveness of this simple exercise. One coaching factor that is often overlooked, though, is the significance of the landing. This represents a force-absorption stimulus similar to high-level plyometrics, although this is rarely considered in

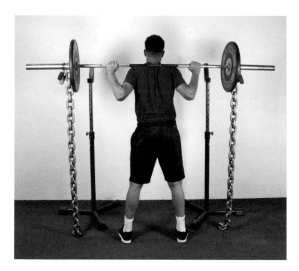

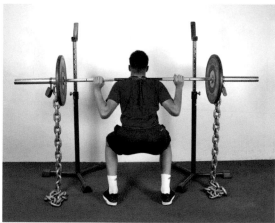

Chain Squats

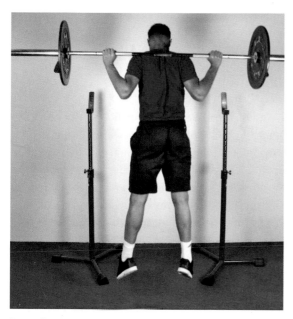

Jump Squats

training. Coaches should be acutely aware that they have the option of using a box to jump onto. The inclusion or exclusion of this intervention will have a profound effect on the total stress sustained by the player in a session (which can obviously be a good or a bad thing).

In the past, a lot of attention has been paid to finding the loading which elicits the highest mechanical power output (incidentally, the answer in jump squats is zero load). However, this is possibly a somewhat misguided pursuit. Rather than there being a 'magical number' which gives the ultimate outcome, power outputs typically show a relatively flat parabola as the load goes up and the jump height reduces. More pertinently though, we need to go back to essential physics and remember that power is a product of force and velocity. Changing the load on the bar allows us to shift the balance between these two elements. Therefore, if we have a player, say a big central

defender, who has lots of force but little velocity, then surely it makes sense to work with lighter loads? Similarly, the reverse would apply with a very speed-dominant player who lacked absolute force generation. Finally, it is likely that it is more effective to work across a range of loadings to achieve a variety of stimuli, rather than looking for the magic number and sticking with it religiously.

Olympic Lifts

Much like the jump squat, the core added value of the Olympic lifts to a football S&C programme is the opportunity to develop a loaded triple extension. There is also the potential for additional athletic gain in the form of coordination, strength and mobility. Unlike the majority of gym-based exercises, the Olympic lifts are inherently explosive and demand a continued acceleration. This makes them a natural fit for sports performance enhancement. The fact that there is a clear outcome in terms of success or failure also makes them appealing to coaches. The desire to improve a personal best in a lift taps into the natural competitiveness of players and helps ensure maximal effort and application.

For some reason, the coaching process often begins with the power clean. While this is less demanding than the power snatch in terms of mobility, it is arguably technically harder. If all things were equal though, I would recommend the power snatch as the better of the two for developing explosiveness as it is far harder to 'muscle' though the lift and rely on upper-body strength. Maybe an even more underused exercise is the jerk. This has the potential to generate huge amounts of torque about the knee, and is a more specific action to running and jumping. The reality though, and reason for its limited use, is that players often lack the upper-body strength to control the loads required to elicit these benefits.

However, for the creative S&C coach, the investment in a set of jerk blocks may help the development of a power-training system that is a little different from the traditional.

The coaching process of the technical aspect of Olympic lifts is clearly crucial, as the movements are not simplistic or naturally occurring. There are many approaches which can be used effectively to this end, much of which is a matter of personal philosophy and what works for you and your players. A key question surrounds whether a top–down or bottom–up approach is taken. A bottom–up approach begins with the start position for a power clean or power snatch from the floor, and progressively builds elements from there. The top–down approach begins with the hang position and moves towards the full lift over time. Traditional weightlifting coaches tend to begin from the floor. This is entirely logical, as their end goal will always be to complete the full lift. However, in an S&C setting we simply need to achieve our loaded triple extension (i.e. the second pull following the hang position). Anything else is a bonus. Therefore my approach, particularly with coaching time-limited football players, would be to start with the simplest form of the lift. This may be something as simple as a hang pull (i.e. jumping and shrugging with a bar in the hands).

Plyometrics & Isometrics

If the large concentric power production seen in jump squats and Olympic lifts is well-suited to acceleration, then alternatives are required to target eccentric strength, stiffness and reactivity required for top-speed running and changes of direction.

It may surprise some that we are discussing plyometrics and isometrics within the same breath, given that the former is characterised by highly explosive, dynamic actions, whereas the latter involves no movement at all. However, both are highly effective at enhancing mechanical stability (i.e. the ability to resist yielding against landing force).

We have already discussed in Chapter 11 how much, if not all, of the plyometric load required may be contained within normal training. Similarly it is important to understand that to get a plyometric stimulus in the form of large impacts and short contacts does not always have to look like an 'exercise'. Sprints, changes of direction and football-related jumping all provide an excellent stimulus in a highly specific manner. However, if you wish to pursue a more traditional approach to plyometrics, or are constrained to the weight room, then there are several factors to consider.

The nature of the exercise can be defined by a number of variables. These include unilateral versus bilateral, vertical versus horizontal movement and ballistic versus rebound. Within these broad categories there are countless exercises that do not need to be listed here. Given that traditional plyometric exercises are inherently less mechanically specific than the naturally occurring football actions that we have already discussed, the key consideration becomes selecting the appropriate intensity level. Essentially the intensity is determined by the highest levels of force sustained during the exercise, with some consideration also given to the level of technical difficulty. Just as novice coaches tend to load the bar too quickly when coaching resistance-training sessions, the temptation with plyometrics is to advance an exercise too soon. To avoid this trap requires patience from the coach and player, and a good eye in the former. It is easy to achieve the illusion of control and balance in

Table 15.1	Plyometric Coaching Fundamentals
Horizontal	**Vertical**
Torso perpendicular to ground	Torso slightly in front of hip
Hip and pelvis stable	Hips, knees and ankles extending in that order
Femur, tib & fib, hip and ankle all perpendicular at stance	Dorsi-flexed ankles
Flat-/mid-foot contact	Flat-foot contact
Single-arm shift for 1-legged, double arm for 2-legged	Double-arm shift with rapid recovery speed of arms

plyometrics by powering through. However, doing so limits the potential gains and significantly heightens the injury risk.

While each exercise naturally has its own nuances, there are several key principles which if understood will allow effective coaching no matter which movement is being performed. These are summarised in Table 15.1.

In terms of volumes of plyometric training, typical recommendations are around 100–120 contacts per session. My view is that while this is appropriate for track-and-field athletes, it is overly conservative for non-strength and power athletes as the intensities achieved are dramatically lower. However, this is unlikely to be an issue in a football environment, as plyometrics will most likely form only a small component of the training. Given the need to accommodate several other forms of training, and the naturally occurring plyometric activity from football sessions and running, I would suggest volumes far lower than this. A typical example may be the use of a drop jump as part of a complex in a gym

session. This is likely to mean around 15–25 contacts (e.g. 3 × 5 reps up to 5 × 5 reps). This relatively small volume will still represent a significant increase in training stress.

Traditionally, whole-body isometric exercises do not tend to feature commonly in training programmes. However, there are a number of advantages to this way of working, which suggest that they should feature more heavily. As we have discussed, they can be equally as effective in improving tendon stiffness and explosive qualities as plyometrics. Unlike plyometrics though, the potentially negative stress of landing impact is removed. This is highly appealing to a football S&C coach, for whom accumulated mechanical stress is likely to represent the ceiling for tolerable training. If a greater training stimulus can be achieved without taking up some of a player's weekly load tolerance, then this should be pursued.

The downside to isometric exercises is that they are generally more elaborate to set up than traditional exercises. However, in recent years, isometric-force testing has become very popular

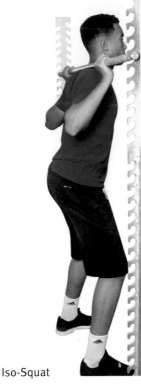

Iso-Squat

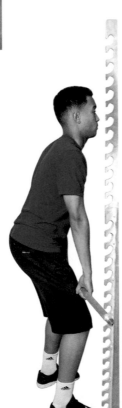

Iso-Pull

within S&C circles. This has led to readily available equipment for the set-up and measurement of isometric work. Customised stands, such as those shown here, are designed specifically to hold the bar in a secure position so that players can exert a maximal effort safely and confidently. These racks also allow for fairly precise adjustment of height so that it is easy to test at a specific joint angle across players of varying heights, without hugely time-consuming adjustments. Typically these are fitted to a lifting platform, which incorporates a force plate. This is an important detail as the force plate not only provides a method of measurement of force for testing purposes but also, crucially, gives real-time feedback as to the level of exertion of the player during training. It is human nature that without any form of feedback players will not be fully motivated to provide the maximal exertion required to get the maximum benefit from this work. The popularity of isometric testing over repetition maximums, particularly in rugby, comes from the fact that technical failure is no longer an issue and so it is possible to get a measure much more representative of pure force production rather than ability in a given lift.

The most popular examples of an isometric exercise for performance enhancement are the iso-squat and the iso-pull (shown left). The iso-squat has the advantage that it probably represents the kinematic action of sprinting and jumping better than the iso-pull. However, it is important that athletes are free from spinal injury, and are both confident and practised at placing a maximal load through their spine before attempting all-out efforts. The issue of specificity in the pull can be overcome somewhat by taking a more upright pulling position with the torso behind the bar. The use of lifting straps is also important in this lift to avoid it becoming simply a test of grip strength.

Finally, because there are no repetitions as such in this type of work, coaches must give consideration to the length of each exertion. This provides a significant amount of freedom in programming. For example, if we wish to accumulate 25s of time under tension during a set, this can be divided up in all manner of ways, e.g. 5 × 5s efforts, 8 × 3s efforts, etc. Manipulating the variables in this way allows for variety of stimulus, even when the intensity and total volume remain the same.

15.4 Conditioning Systems

As we learnt in Chapter 4, a key component of an injury-prevention system is increased tissue tolerance. Unlike the movement focus taken so far within this chapter, it now becomes appropriate to talk in terms of the specific tissues, i.e. a particular muscle group, tendon, etc., which we wish to target. The following section aims to provide more than a list of exercises for a given muscle group. Instead, we can explore what the functional challenges to each area are, and the most effective methods of eliciting the appropriate adaptations.

Hamstrings

In Chapter 6 we outlined a comprehensive hamstring-injury prevention system which considers a multi-factorial model of the issue. Improving the capacity of the muscle is simply one of five key strands to this system. Therefore it is important to reiterate that what follows is simply a guide to some of the most suitable tools in achieving this specific outcome.

I like to loosely categorise hamstring exercises as: **low intensity–high function**, **basic conditioning** and **high intensity–high function**.

Motor-patterning work for hamstring control can be developed with little tissue stress through **low**

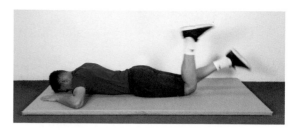

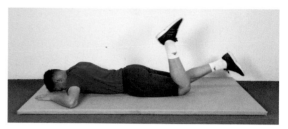

Flutters

intensity–high function work. Exercises such as flutters (above) replicate the functional demand on the hamstrings to decelerate knee extension very rapidly. The forces involved are relatively low and consequently players can tolerate high volumes without much fatigue. This is also a result of the fact that the time under tension in the muscle is very low. Therefore the primary adaptation occurs within the nervous system rather than the tissues themselves. Similar effects can be achieved through exercises such as C-drills, and even through pushing on a scooter. In these two examples the hamstrings are required to resist knee extension isometrically while producing extension of the hip, just like in running. These are all excellent end-stage rehab exercises for hamstrings when there is a need to work in function specific ways, but tolerance of sprint running may still be compromised.

Basic conditioning exercises are characterised by the fact that, as a reversal of the bias in the low intensity–high function exercise above, the

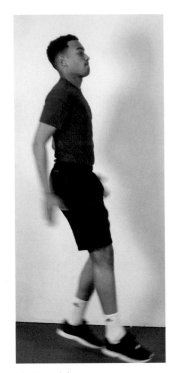
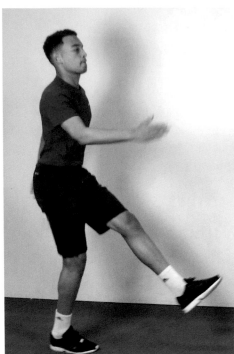
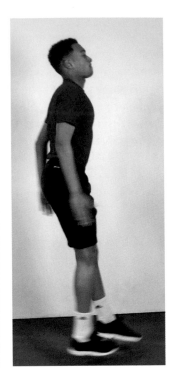

Flutter Kicks

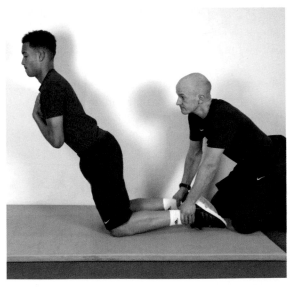
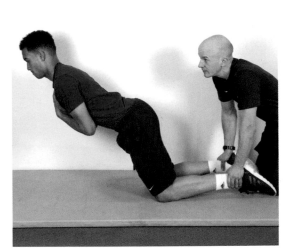

Nordic Curls

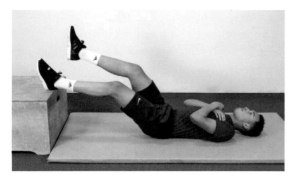

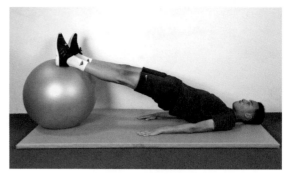

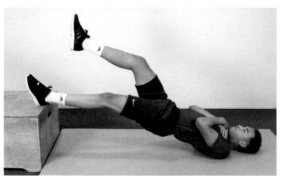

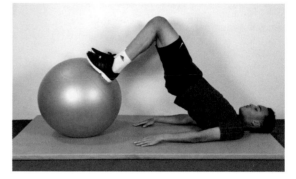

Hamstring Bridge

Swiss Ball Hamstring Curl

emphasis is very much on simply stressing the muscle to achieve an adaptive training stress. These can be subdivided into hip-extension and knee-flexion exercises. This is not intended as an attempt to achieve motor specificity, but simply a reflection of the fact that the differing movements will bring about a shift in emphasis between the medial and lateral hamstrings. Consideration should also be given to unilateral versus bilateral choices, as well as open- versus closed-chain movements. There are almost countless examples which can be drawn upon. The exercise selection should be based upon the kinematic factors we have just discussed, in order to target the desired tissues. Thereafter, the choice centres around matching an exercise to the desired intensity. The highest levels of muscular stress are typically seen in eccentric exercises such as

Nordic curls. It should be noted that in addition to the high-training stimulus achieved in these movements, there also appears to be the capacity to lengthen the fascicles and increase the optimum length of the muscle (this is a good thing). Therefore the adaptation is not only greater but also different.

High intensity–high function exercises combine the best of each of the former categories. Sprint running is perhaps the best example of this category. Another exercise which has gained popularity recently is the so-called Bosch-Hamstring exercise, named after its creator, Frans Bosch (see page 168). This places large isometric stresses on the hamstrings in a position similar to that during ground contact in sprinting. Other very useful options include the step-down lunge, which

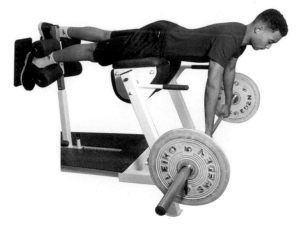

Bosch Hamstrings

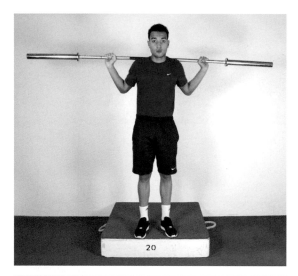

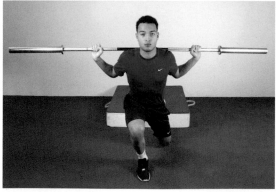

Step-Down Lunge

calls for rapid eccentric deceleration in a whole-body movement, and single-leg RDLs which demand good control of the pelvis throughout the movement.

Calves

When we talk of strengthening the calf complex, we are very much concerned with the muscle-tendon unit (MTU) as a whole rather than simply the muscle in isolation. The importance of the health of MTU as a system in regard to reduction of injury to both muscle and tendon is well documented.

As with the hamstrings, there are several distinct categories which I have found it useful to group calf training into. **Proprioception and balance** work requires high levels of activation of the calf musculature (particularly the peroneals). However, this has the added benefit of developing proprioception about the ankle, and therefore potentially reducing the burden on the calf during training and competition activity. Barefoot work, particularly during warm-ups, can be an excellent way of incorporating this type of activity, and carries the added benefit of developing the

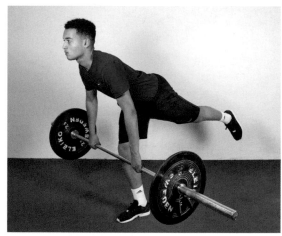

Single-Leg RDL

intrinsic musculature of the feet, which is often overlooked in conditioning programmes. Possibly the most efficient and simple method of gaining this type of training stimulus is through the use of sand as a training surface. There are few more effective calf workouts than multi-directional running barefoot on nicely churned-up sand.

The second category of calf work is the more traditional view of movements that are essentially **loaded plantar flexion**, such as calf raises. As most S&C coaches will be aware, these need to be performed with both a straight leg and a bent leg in order to effectively target both gastrocnemius and soleus. Naturally, while not strictly part of the calf, tibialis anterior should also be trained through dorsi-flexion movements such as toe raises. During these types of exercises, which are directly targeted at tissue adaptation, time under tension is key. Therefore it is important that a controlled tempo is held, rather than a bouncing-type action. Eccentric calf raises, or heel drops, are a popular prescription towards the goal of increasing tissue quality in the Achilles tendon. While this is a perfectly legitimate strategy, it is often poorly executed due to insufficient load. Remember, there is nothing inherently magical about the eccentric phase. The value comes from the fact that greater maximal eccentric loads can be tolerated than through a concentric action. However, if a set of eccentrics is performed with a load that the player could perform through a normal con-ecc motion, then nothing has been gained. Very high loads can be taken through the ankle, and so to achieve a genuine eccentric overload a barbell, preferably a safety squat bar, or a leg press are the best options. A 10kg dumbbell will certainly not do the job!

Finally, the need to develop **stiffness and reactivity** through the calf and ankle must not be

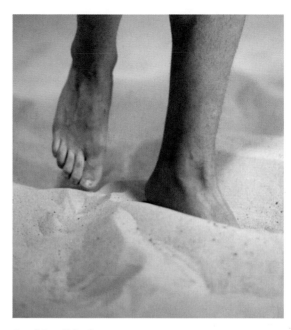

Sand Conditioning

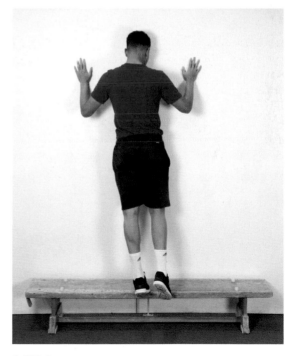

Calf Raise

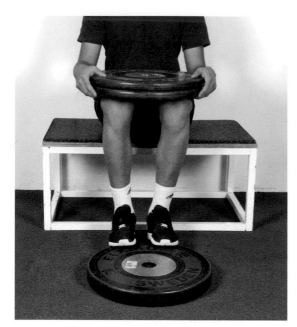

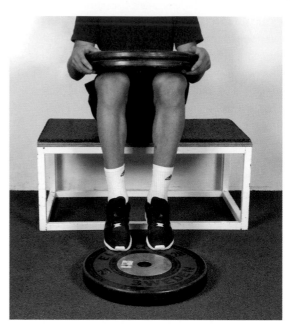

Seated Calf Raise

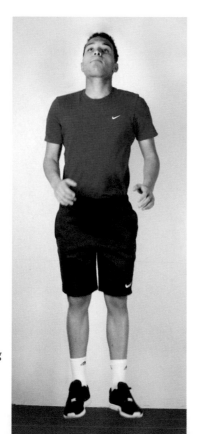

Rebound Jumping

forgotten. This involves developing the nervous system as well as the tissues. There is a requisite need to build the skill of pre-activation prior to ground contact in order to keep the ankle stable and transfer force effectively. Again, sprint running is a highly effective method of achieving this stimulus and is clearly highly specific. As we have learnt earlier in this chapter, isometric work through the calf is also effective for producing these qualities. Plyometrics are of course a natural choice. While ankle stiffness is required in pretty much all lower-body plyometrics, exercises which involve minimal hip and knee flexion, such as rebound jumping, are particularly effective.

Gluteals

Classification of glute exercises is perhaps a somewhat more simplistic task than with hamstrings and calves (as these are biarticular whereas the glutes are not). Glute work can be thought of on a continuum of functionality. As

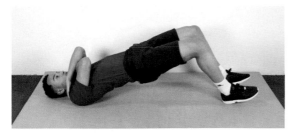

Glute Bridge

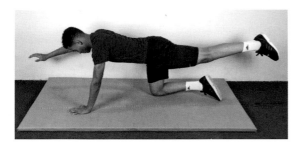

Superman

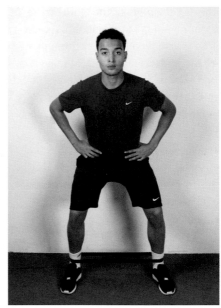

Band Walks

many people are not comfortable with the term 'functional', it may be better to think in terms of isolated activity versus coordinated activity. Unlike the calf and the hamstring, strain injury to the glutes is relatively uncommon. However, a lack of capacity in this area can lead to excessive burden in other muscles such as the hamstrings, or a lack of control of the knee.

Training culture boasts a large range of **low-level, isolated glute work,** which is commonly prescribed by physiotherapists. This often follows a diagnosis that the muscle group is 'underactive'. Therefore the focus of these low-intensity exercises is to promote activation. Classic examples include the glute bridge, band walks and superman.

These exercises are entirely fit for task, however, once the player has learnt to recruit the musculature correctly without compensations, then these need to be loaded further to provide an overload stimulus. I have found that smart manipulation of training variables is often lacking in prescription of this type of work, with coaches remaining static on the same exercises, with the same loading and the same prescription. This type of stale programming is endemic in prehab sessions, and not only results in a lack of training gains but also surely contributes to player apathy and lack of interest. Competitive athletes thrive on progression! The glutes are a powerful muscle group and can tolerate high loadings. Therefore exercises such as the barbell bridge (below) can be used to provide a very high stimulus.

Ultimately, there comes a need to incorporate increases in glute strength into a functional pattern. Athletics drills such as hurdle walk-throughs and A-Marching are excellent for incorporating the glutes into a complex motor pattern. The key to both of these challenges is to 'keep the hips high' and avoid 'sitting down'.

Essentially, this is the ability of the glute on the standing side to remain in extension through the movement. This is achieved primarily through recruitment of the gluteus maximus. Equally importantly the gluteus medius and minimus must work to stabilise the hip laterally, and avoid a Trendelenburg movement (hip kicking out). A less complex but higher-load integrated glute challenge can also be found in the humble squat. A good, hip-dominant squat is an excellent way to train the glutes to produce a forceful hip extension in a coordinated pattern (and therefore reduce load on the hamstrings).

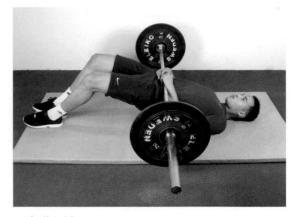

Barbell Bridge

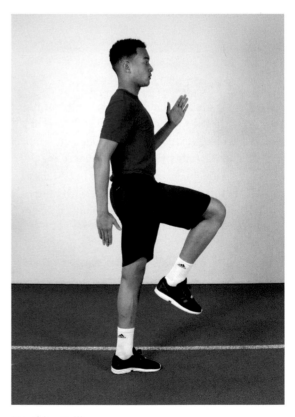

Marching Drill

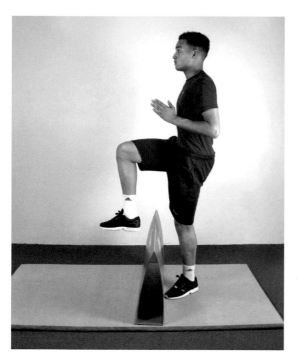
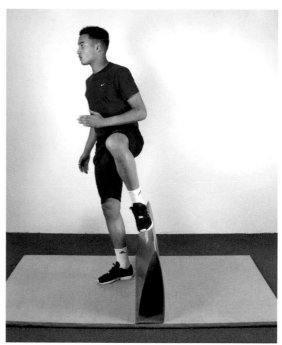
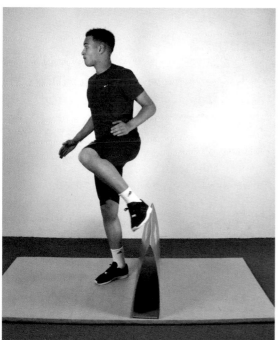
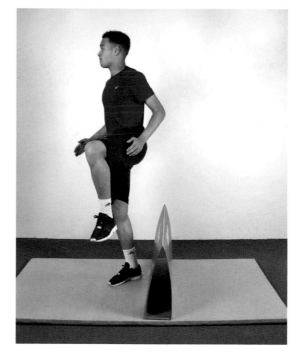

Hurdle March

further reading

Chapter 1
Ackerman, P. L. (2014), 'Nonsense, common sense, and science of expert performance: Talent and individual differences', in *Intelligence*. Elsevier.

Chapter 2
Anderson, C. and D. Sally (2013), *The Numbers Game – Why Everything You Know About Football is Wrong*. Penguin.

Bradley, P. S., et al. (2013), 'Match performance and physical capacity of players in the top three competitive standards of English professional soccer', in *Human Movement Science*. **32**(4): pp. 808–21. Elsevier.

Helgerud, J., et al. (2001), 'Aerobic endurance training improves soccer performance', in *Medicine & Science in Sports & Exercise*. **33**(11): pp. 1925–31. American College of Sports Medicine.

Chapter 3
Cook, C. J. and Crewther, B. T. (2012a), 'Changes in salivary testosterone concentrations and subsequent voluntary squat performance following the presentation of short video clips', in *Hormones & Behavior*, **61**: pp. 17–22. Elsevier.

Cook, C. J. and Crewther, B. T. (2012b), 'The effects of different pre-game motivational interventions on athlete free hormonal state and subsequent performance in professional rugby union matches', in *Physiology & Behavior*, **106**: pp. 683–88. Elsevier.

Spiering, B. (2012), *Maintaining Peak Physical Performance*. Presented at UKSCA Conference.

Chapter 4
Aagaard, P. (2012), *Hyperactivation of Myogenic Satellite Cells with Blood Flow Restricted*

Exercise, presented at the 8th International Conference on Strength Training. Oslo.

Baker, D., S. Nance, and M. Moore (2001), 'The load that maximizes the average mechanical power output during jump squats in power-trained athletes', in *Journal of Strength & Conditioning Research*. **15**(1): pp. 92–7. LWW Journals.

Bosch, F. (2013) 'Basic Motor Properties', in *EIS CPD*.

Bosch, F. and R. Klomp (2005), *Running: Biomechanics and exercise physiology in practice*. Elsevier Churchill Livingstone.

Burgess, K. E., et al. (2007), 'Plyometric vs. isometric training influences on tendon properties and muscle output', in *Journal of Strength & Conditioning Research*. **21**(3): pp. 986–9. LWW Journals.

Cook, J. L., et al. (2004), 'Neovascularization and pain in abnormal patellar tendons of active jumping athletes', in *Clinical Journal of Sports Medicine*. **14**(5): pp. 296–9. LWW Journals.

Croisier, J. L., et al. (2002), 'Hamstring muscle strain recurrence and strength performance disorders', in *American Journal of Sports Medicine*. **30**(2): pp. 199–203. Sage.

Gabriel, D. A., G. Kamen and G. Frost (2006), 'Neural adaptations to resistive exercise: mechanisms and recommendations for training practices', in *Sports Medicine*. **36**(2): pp. 133–49. Springer International Publisher.

Kidgell, D. and A. Pearce (2011), 'What has transcranial magnetic stimulation taught us about neural adaptations to strength training? a brief review', in *Journal of Strength & Conditioning Research*. **25**(11). LWW Journals.

Kon, M., et al. (2012), 'Effects of low-intensity resistance exercise under acute systemic hypoxia on hormonal responses', in *Journal of Strength & Conditioning Research*. **26**(3). LWW Journals.

Kongsgaard, M., et al. (2007), 'Region specific patellar tendon hypertrophy in humans following resistance training', in *Acta Physiologiae Plantarum* (Oxf). **191**(2): pp. 111–21. Springer International Publisher.

Kubo, K., et al. (2006), 'Effects of isometric squat training on the tendon stiffness and jump performance', in *European Journal of Applied Physiology*. **96**(3): pp. 305–14. American Physiological Society.

Laursen, J. B., D. M. Bertelsen and L. B. Andersen (2014), 'The effectiveness of exercise interventions to prevent sports injuries: a systematic review and meta-analysis of randomised controlled trials', in *British Journal of Sports Medicine*. **48**(11): pp. 871–77. BJM Journals.

Lederman, E. (2010), 'The myth of core stability', in *Journal of Bodywork & Movement Therapies*. **14**. Elsevier.

Miller, B. F., et al. (2005), 'Coordinated collagen and muscle protein synthesis in human patella tendon and quadriceps muscle after exercise', in *Journal of Physiology*. **567**(Pt 3): pp. 1021–33. Wiley.

Myer, G. D., et al. (2011), 'Did the NFL Lockout Expose the Achilles Heel of Competitive Sports?', in *Journal of Orthopaedic & Sports Physical Therapy*. **41**(10).

Myers, T. (2008), *Anatomy Trains: Myofascial Meridians for Manual and Movement Therapists*, 2nd edn. Churchill Livingstone.

Nilsson, J. and A. Thorstensson (1989), 'Ground reaction forces at different speeds of human walking and running', in *Acta Physiologica Scandinavica*. **136**(2): pp. 217–27. Wiley.

Nishimura, A., et al. (2010), 'Hypoxia increases muscle hypertrophy induced by resistance training', in *International Journal of Sports Physiology and Performance*. **5**: pp. 497–508. Human Kinetics.

Reeves, G.V., et al. (2006), 'Comparison of hormone responses following light resistance exercise with partial vascular occlusion and moderately difficult resistance exercise without occlusion', in *Journal of Applied Physiology*. **101**(6): p. 1616–22. American Physiological Society.

Rosenblatt, B. (2012), *The Effect of Low Load Blood Flow Restricted Resistance Training in Rehabilitation of Elite Athletes*, presented at the 8th International Conference on Strength Training. Oslo.

Rosenblatt, B. (2013), 'Training Tendons', in *Bath EIS CPD Day*: Bath.

Starrett, K. and G. Cardoza (2013), *Becoming a Supple Leopard: The Ultimate Guide to Resolving Pain, Preventing Injury, and Optimizing Athletic Performance*. Victory Belt Publishing Inc.

Takarada, Y., et al. (2000), 'Rapid increase in plasma growth hormone after low-intensity resistance exercise with vascular occlusion', in *Journal of Applied Physiology*. **88**(1): pp. 61–5. American Physiological Society.

Takarada, Y., H. Takazawa, and N. Ishii (2000), 'Applications of vascular occlusion diminish disuse atrophy of knee extensor muscles', in *Medicine & Science in Sports & Exercise*. **32**(12): pp. 2035–9. American Journal of Sports Medicine.

Wernborn, M. (2012), *Blood Flow Restricted Resistance Exercise: Possible Stimuli and Signaling Pathways*, presented at the 8th International Conference on Strength Training. Oslo.

Wulf, G., C. Shea and R. Lewthwaite (2010), 'Motor skill learning and performance: a review of influential factors', in *Medical Education*. **44**: pp. 75–84. Wiley.

Chapter 5

Anderson, C. and D. Sally (2013), *The Numbers Game – Why Everything You Know About Football is Wrong*. Penguin.

Bennell, K., et al. (1998), 'Isokinetic strength testing does not predict hamstring injury in Australian Rules footballers', in *British Journal of Sports Medicine*. **32**: pp. 309–14. BMJ Journals.

Bradley, P. S., et al. (2013), 'Match performance and physical capacity of players in the top three competitive standards of English professional soccer', in *Human Movement Science*. **32**(4): pp. 808–21. Elsevier.

Demoulin, C., et al. (2006), 'Spinal muscle evaluation using the Sorensen test: a critical appraisal of the literature', in *Joint Bone Spine*. **73**(1): pp. 43–50. Elsevier.

Freckleton, G., J. Cook and T. Pizzari (2013), 'The predictive validity of a single leg bridge test for hamstring injuries in Australian Rules Football Players', in *British Journal of Sports Medicine*. BMJ Journals.

Gribble, P. A., J. Hertel and P. Plisky (2012), 'Using the Star Excursion Balance Test to assess dynamic postural-control deficits and outcomes in lower extremity injury: a literature and systematic review', in *Journal of Athletic Training*. **47**(3): pp. 339–57.

Hawkins, R. D., et al. (2001), 'The association football medical research programme: an audit of injuries in professional football', in *British Journal of Sports Medicine*. **35**(1): pp. 43–7. BMJ Journals.

Hébert-Losier, K., et al. (2009), 'Scientific bases and clinical utilisation of the calf-raise test', in *Physical Therapy in Sport*. **10**(4): pp. 142–9. Elsevier.

Henry, J. C. and C. Kaeding (2001), 'Neuromuscular differences between male and female athletes', in *Current Women's Health Reports*. **1**(3): pp. 241–4.

Kahneman, D. (2011), *Thinking, fast and slow*. Macmillan.

Konrad, P., K. Schmitz and A. Denner (2001), 'Neuromuscular Evaluation of Trunk-Training Exercises', in *Journal of Athletic Training*. **36**(2): pp. 109–18.

Le Gall, F., et al. (2006), 'Incidence of injuries in elite French youth soccer players: a 10-season study', in *American Journal of Sports Medicine*. **34**(6): pp. 928–38. Sage.

Mallo, J. and A. Dellal (2012), 'Injury risk in professional football players with special reference to the playing position and training periodization', in *Journal of Sports Medicine & Physical Fitness*. **52**(6): pp. 631–8. Minerva Medici.

Noya Salces, J., et al. (2014), 'Epidemiology of injuries in First Division Spanish football', in *Journal of Sports Science*, pp. 1–8. Taylor & Francis.

Chapter 6

Aagaard, P. (2009), *Prevention of Hamstring Injury* – UKA Presentation.

Bosch, F. (2012), *Positive running, a model for high speed running*, presented at the International Festival of Athletics Coaching. Scotland.

Brockett, C., D. Morgan and U. Proske (2001), 'Human hamstring muscles adapt to eccentric exercise by changing optimum length', in *Medicine and Science in Sports and Exercise*. **33**(5). Wolters Kluwer.

Brukner, P., et al. (2012), 'Recurrent hamstring muscle injury: applying the limited evidence in the professional football setting with a seven-point programme', in *British Journal of Sports Medicine*. BMJ Journals.

Croisier, J. L. (2004), 'Factors associated with recurrent hamstring injuries', in *Sports Medicine*. **34**(10): pp. 681–95. Springer International Publisher.

Croisier, J. L., et al. (2002), 'Hamstring muscle strain recurrence and strength performance disorders', in *American Journal of Sports Medicine*. **30**(2): pp. 199–203. Sage.

Marshall, P. W., et al. (2014), *Hamstring Muscle Fatigue and Central Motor Output during a Simulated Soccer Match*. PLOS One. **9**(7): p. e102753.

Mendiguchia, J., E. Alentorn-Geli, and M. Brughelli (2012), 'Hamstring strain injuries: are we heading in the right direction?', in *British Journal of Sports Medicine*. **46**(2). BMJ Journals.

Schollhorn, W. (2012), *Differential Learning*, EIS Presentation.

Sherry, M. and T. Best (2004), 'A Comparison of 2 Rehabilitation Programs in the Treatment of Acute Hamstring Strains', in *Journal of Orthopaedic & Sports Physical Therapy*. **34**(3).

Small, K., et al. (2009), 'Effect of Timing of Eccentric Hamstring Strengthening Exercises During Soccer Training: Implications for Muscle Fatigability', in *Journal of Strength & Conditioning Research*. **23**(4). LWW Journals.

Woods, C., et al. (2004), 'The Football Association Medical Research Programme: an audit of injuries in professional football – analysis of hamstring injuries', in *British Journal of Sports Medicine*. **38**. BMJ Journals.

Chapter 7

Allen, J. and S. Butler (2010), 'The groin in sport', in *Sports Rehabilitation and Injury Prevention*, P. Comfort and E. Abrahamson, eds. Wiley-Blackwell.

Coughlan, G. F., et al. (2014), 'Normative Adductor Squeeze Test Values in Elite Junior Rugby Union Players', in *Clinical Journal of Sports Medicine*. LWW Journals.

Delahunt, E., et al. (2011), 'Intrarater reliability of the adductor squeeze test in gaelic games athletes', in *Journal of Athletic Training*. **46**(3): pp. 241–5. NATA Journals.

Hrysomallis, C. (2009), 'Hip adductors' strength, flexibility, and injury risk', in *Journal of Strength & Conditioning Research*. **23**(5): pp. 1514–17. LWW Journals.

Maffey, L. and C. Emery (2007), 'What are the risk factors for groin strain injury in sport? A systematic review of the literature', in *Sports Medicine*. **37**(10): pp. 881–94. Springer International Publisher.

McGill, S. (2009), *Ultimate Back Fitness and Performance*, 4th edn. Wabuno.

Myers, T. (2008), *Anatomy Trains: Myofascial Meridians for Manual and Movement Therapists*, 2nd edn. Churchill Livingstone.

Chapter 8

Clark, N. and L. Herrington (2010), 'The knee', in *Sports Rehabilitation and Injury Prevention*, P. Comfort and E. Abrahamson, eds. pp. 407–64. Wiley-Blackwell.

Gu, Y., et al. (2014), 'Effects of different unstable sole construction on kinematics and muscle activity of lower limb', in *Human Movement Science*. **36C**: pp. 46–57. Elsevier.

Hawkins, R.D., et al. (2001), 'The association football medical research programme: an audit of injuries in professional football', in *British Journal of Sports Medicine*. **35**(1): pp. 43–7. BMJ Journals.

Hart, J. M., et al. (2010), 'Quadriceps activation following knee injuries: a systematic review', in *Journal of Athletic Training*. **45**(1): pp. 87–97. NATA Journals.

Hartmann, H., K. Wirth and M. Klusemann (2013), 'Analysis of the load on the knee joint and vertebral column with changes in squatting depth and weight load', in *Sports Medicine*. **43**(10): pp. 993–1008. Springer International Publisher.

Hewett, T. E., et al. (2005), 'Biomechanical measures of neuromuscular control and valgus loading of the knee predict anterior cruciate ligament injury risk in female athletes: a prospective study', in *American Journal of Sports Medicine*. **33**(4): pp. 492–501. Sage.

Noyes, F. R. and S. D. Barber Westin (2012), 'Anterior cruciate ligament injury prevention training in female athletes: a systematic review of injury reduction and results of athletic performance tests', in *Sports Health*. **4**(1): pp. 36–46. Sage.

Orchard, J. W., et al. (2013), 'Comparison of injury incidences between football teams playing in different climatic regions', in *Open Access Journal of Sports Medicine*. **4**: pp. 251–60. Dove Medical Press.

Powers, C. M. (2010), 'The influence of abnormal hip mechanics on knee injury: a biomechanical perspective', in *Journal of Orthopaedic & Sports Physical Therapy*. **40**(2): pp. 42–51.

Sale, D. G. (1988), 'Neural adaptation to resistance training', in *Medicine & Science in Sports & Exercise*. **20**(5 Supplement): pp. S135–45. American College of Sports Medicine.

Chapter 9

Anderson, C. and D. Sally (2013), *The Numbers Game – Why Everything You Know About Football is Wrong*. Penguin.

Mendez-Villanueva, A., et al. (2011), 'Does on-field sprinting performance in young soccer players depend on how fast they can run or how fast they do run?', in *Journal of Strength & Conditioning Research*. **25**(9): pp. 2634–8. LWW Journals.

van Gaal, L., F. Hoek and L. Lainz (2012). *Barcelona Philosophy*. Available from: http://www.slideshare.net/coachingtech/barcelonaphilosophy1.

Chapter 10

Bosch, F. and R. Klomp (2005), *Running: Biomechanics and exercise physiology in practice*. Elsevier Churchill Livingstone.

Buchheit, M. and P. Laursen (2013), 'High-intensity interval training, solutions to the programming puzzle', in *Sports Medicine*. **43**. Springer International Publisher.

Cronin, J. B. and K.T. Hansen (2005), 'Strength and power predictors of sports speed', in *Journal of Strength & Conditioning Research*. **19**(2): pp. 349–57. LWW Journals.

Faude, O., T. Koch and T. Meyer (2012), 'Straight sprinting is the most frequent action in goal situations in professional football', in *Journal of Sports Sciences*. **30**. Taylor & Francis.

Mann, R. (2011), *The Mechanics of Sprinting and Hurdling*. CreateSpace Independent Publishing Platform.

Mendez-Villanueva, A., et al. (2011), 'Does on-field sprinting performance in young soccer players depend on how fast they can run or how fast they do run?', in *Journal of Strength & Conditioning Research*. **25**(9): pp. 2634–8. LWW Journals.

Starrett, K. and G. Cardoza (2013), *Becoming a Supple Leopard: The Ultimate Guide to Resolving Pain, Preventing Injury, and Optimizing Athletic Performance*. Victory Belt Publishing Inc.

Williams, A. M. (2000), 'Perceptual skill in soccer: implications for talent identification and development', in *Journal of Sports Science*. **18**(9): pp. 737–50. Taylor & Francis.

Wisloff, U., et al. (2004), 'Strong correlation of maximal squat strength with sprint performance and vertical jump height in elite soccer players', in *British Journal of Sports Medicine*. **38**(3): pp. 285–8. BMJ Journals.

Wulf, G. (2007), *Methods of enhancing motor learning – A review of 10 years of research*. Bewegung und Training.

Wulf, G., C. Shea, and R. Lewthwaite (2010), 'Motor skill learning and performance: a review of influential factors', in *Medical Education*. **44**: pp. 75–84. Wiley.

Young, M. (2013) *Science of Speed*. Available from: http://www.slideshare.net/hpcsport/2013-pres-royal-college-of-chiropractors-sports-sciences-neuromechanics-of-speed#.

Young, W., B. McLean and J. Ardagna (1995), 'Relationship between strength qualities and sprinting performance', in *Journal of Sports Medicine & Physical Fitness*. **35**(1): pp. 13–19. Minerva Medica.

Chapter 11

Barr, M. J., et al. (2014), 'Transfer effect of strength and power training to the sprinting kinematics of international rugby players', in *Journal of Strength & Conditioning Research*. **28**(9): pp. 2585–96. LWW Journals.

Beaven, C. M., N. D. Gill, and C. J. Cook (2008), 'Salivary testosterone and cortisol responses in professional rugby players after four resistance exercise protocols', in *Journal of Strength & Conditioning Research*. **22**(2): pp. 426–32. LWW Journals.

Cook, C. J., C. M. Beaven and L. P. Kilduff (2013), 'Three weeks of eccentric training combined with overspeed exercises enhances power and running speed performance gains in trained athletes', in *Journal of Strength & Conditioning Research*. **27**(5): pp. 1280–6. LWW Journals.

Cormie, P. (2011), *The Influence of Strength on Muscular Power (Part 1)*. UKSCA Presentation.

Cormie, P. (2011), *The Influence of Strength on Muscular Power (Part 2)*. UKSCA Presentation.

Hartmann, H., et al. (2012), 'Influence of squatting depth on jumping performance', in *Journal of Strength & Conditioning Research*. **26**(12): pp. 3243–61. LWW Journals.

Jarvis, M. M., P. Graham-Smith, and P. Comfort (2014), 'A Methodological Approach to Quantifying Plyometric Intensity', in *Journal of Strength & Conditioning Research*. LWW Journals.

Spiteri, T., et al. (2013), 'Effect of strength on plant foot kinetics and kinematics during a change of direction task', in *European Journal of Sport Science*. pp. 1–7. Taylor & Francis.

Spiteri, T., et al. (2014), 'The contribution of strength characteristics to change of direction and agility performance in female basketball athletes', in *Journal of Strength & Conditioning Research*. LWW Journals.

Verkoshansky, Y. and M. C. Siff (2009), *Supertraining (Sixth Edition – Expanded Version)*. 6th edn. Ultimate Athletic Concepts.

West, D. J., et al. (2013), 'Effects of resisted sprint training on acceleration in professional rugby union players', in *Journal of Strength & Conditioning Research*. **27**(4): pp. 1014–8. LWW Journals.

Young, M. (2013), *Science of Speed*. Available from: http://www.slideshare.net/hpcsport/2013-pres-royal-college-of-chiropractors-sports-sciences-neuromechanics-of-speed#.

Young, W., B. McLean, and J. Ardagna (1995), 'Relationship between strength qualities and sprinting performance', in *Journal of Sports Medicine & Physical Fitness*. **35**(1): pp. 13–19. Minerva Medica.

Young, W. B. (2006), 'Transfer of strength and power training to sports performance', in *International Journal of Sports Physiology and Performance*. **1**(2): pp. 74–83. Human Kinetics Journals.

Young, W. B., R. James, and I. Montgomery (2002), 'Is muscle power related to running speed with changes of direction?', in *Journal of Sports Medicine & Physical Fitness*. **42**(3): pp. 282–8. Minerva Medica.

Chapter 12

Bronson, P. and A. Merryman (2014), *Top Dog – The Science of Winning & Losing*. Ebury Press.

Carre, J. M. and S. K. Putnam (2010), 'Watching a previous victory produces an increase in testosterone among elite hockey players', in *Psychoneuroendocrinology*. **35**(3): pp. 475–9. Elsevier.

Contreras, B. and B. Schoenfeld (2011), 'To crunch or not to crunch: an evidence-based examination of spinal flexion exercises, their potential risks, and their applicability to program design', in *Strength & Conditioning Journal*. **33**(4): pp. 8–18. LWW Journals.

Cook, C. J. and B. T. Crewther (2012a), 'The effects of different pre-game motivational interventions on athlete free hormonal state and subsequent performance in professional rugby union matches', in *Physiology & Behavior*. **106**(5): pp. 683–8. Elsevier.

Cook, C. J. and B. T. Crewther (2012b), 'Changes in salivary testosterone concentrations and subsequent voluntary squat performance following the presentation of short video clips', in *Hormones & Behavior*. **61**(1): pp. 17–22. Elsevier.

Mann, R. (2011), *The Mechanics of Sprinting and Hurdling*. CreateSpace Independent Publishing Platform.

McGill, S. (2009), *Ultimate Back Fitness and Performance*. 4th edn. Wabuno.

Myers, T. (2008), *Anatomy Trains: Myofascial Meridians for Manual and Movement Therapists*. 2nd edn. Churchill Livingstone.